174.28
H88

DETROIT PUBLIC LIBRARY

W9-CHY-429

CONELY BRANCH LIBRARY
4600 MARTIN
DETROIT, MI 48210
(313) 224-6461

DEC   06
MAY   '08
SEP   04
JAN 06
APR   06
JUN   '05
DEC   '05

HUMAN
EMBRYO
EXPERIMENTATION

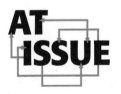

Roman Espejo, *Book Editor*

Daniel Leone, *President*
Bonnie Szumski, *Publisher*
Scott Barbour, *Managing Editor*

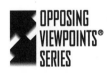

OPPOSING
VIEWPOINTS®
SERIES

GREENHAVEN PRESS
SAN DIEGO, CALIFORNIA

THOMSON
GALE

Detroit • New York • San Diego • San Francisco
Boston • New Haven, Conn. • Waterville, Maine
London • Munich

MAY   2004

No part of this book may be reproduced or used in any form or by any means, electrical, mechanical, or otherwise, including, but not limited to, photocopy, recording, or any information storage and retrieval system, without prior written permission from the publisher.

Library of Congress Cataloging-in-Publication Data

Human embryo experimentation / Roman Espejo, book editor.
    p. cm. — (At issue)
    Includes bibliographical references and index.
    ISBN 0-7377-1284-8 (pbk. : alk. paper) —
   ISBN 0-7377-1285-6 (lib. bdg. : alk. paper)
    1. Embryonic stem cells—Research—Moral and ethical aspects.
    2. Human embryo—Research—Moral and ethical aspects.
    I. Espejo, Roman, 1977– . II. At issue (San Diego, Calif.)

QP277 .H85   2002
174'.28—dc21   2002023637

Copyright © 2002 by Greenhaven Press,
an imprint of The Gale Group
10911 Technology Place, San Diego, CA 92127

Printed in the U.S.A.

Every effort has been made to trace owners of copyrighted material.

CONELY BRANCH

Contents

Page

Introduction   4

1. Embryonic Stem Cell Research Is Beneficial   6
   National Institutes of Health

2. Human Embryo Experimentation Can Be Morally Justifiable   13
   Michael J. Meyer and Lawrence J. Nelson

3. Early Human Embryos Are Not Human Beings   26
   Helga Kuhse and Peter Singer

4. Embryonic Stem Cell Research Should Be Federally Funded   36
   Lawrence S.B. Goldstein

5. Cloning Human Embryos for Therapeutic Purposes Should Be Allowed   39
   Michael D. West

6. Embryonic Stem Cell Research Is Unethical   45
   Center for Bioethics and Human Dignity

7. The Immediate Benefits of Embryonic Stem Cell Research Are Exaggerated   54
   Charles Krauthammer

8. Early Human Embryos Are Human Beings   58
   Andrew Sullivan

9. Cloning Human Embryos for Therapeutic Purposes Should Be Banned   61
   Mae-Wan Ho and Joe Cummins

10. Frozen Embryo Adoption Should Be Encouraged   67
    JoAnn L. Davidson

Organizations to Contact   72

Bibliography   75

Index   77

Introduction

Scientific experiments on human embryos were first initiated for research to develop in vitro fertilization (IVF)—literally "fertilization in glass"—to enable infertile couples to have children. In this procedure, eggs and sperm are taken from a couple and fertilized by scientific means, outside of sexual reproduction. The resulting early staged embryos, or blastocysts, are implanted into the mother's womb with the intent to achieve pregnancy.

Although efforts at in vitro fertilization with animals can be traced back to the late 1800s, it was not until 1965 that IVF technologies were applied to human reproduction. In 1971, researchers Patrick Steptoe, Robert Edwards, and Jean Purdy publicly announced that they had produced the first in vitro human blastocyst. Seven years later, Steptoe and Edwards announced the birth of Louise Brown, the first child to be been born as a result of in vitro fertilization. By the 1980s, IVF became a widely used method of treating both female and male infertility, allowing thousands of infertile couples to raise children biologically related to them.

From the beginning, in vitro fertilization has generated public controversy, especially among those with Christian views of procreation, the sanctity of life, and abortion. For instance, because the egg is fertilized without sexual reproduction, some Christians feel that IVF undermines the sacred act of procreative sexual intercourse between two married individuals. In addition, since several IVF-related practices require the destruction of blastocysts, it contradicts the Christian view that because life begins at the moment of conception, the destruction or abortion of the human embryo is murder. However, while some Christians today adamantly oppose in vitro fertilization, its ability to fulfill the wishes of many couples to have children has broadened the public's acceptance of the procedure.

Couples who elect IVF to negate infertility face both physical and emotional challenges. Success with IVF takes a great deal of patience, persistence, and hope. Because the success rate of IVF is low, many blastocysts are produced at one time. In fact, the vast majority of them are never implanted into a womb. At the discretion of their genetic parents, extra blastocysts are frozen and stored for future use by the couple, discarded, or donated to scientific experimentation.

Human embryo experimentation has been used—and is continuously pursued—to expand our knowledge of the human embryo, improve contraception and fertility treatments, and develop prenatal screening for genetic conditions and abnormalities. But in 1994, Congress prohibited the federal funding of human embryo experimentation that takes place outside the womb. This policy is based on the belief that blastocysts living outside the womb are live human beings and therefore have the right not to be subjected to experimentation without their consent.

In recent years, the debate over human embryo experimentation has intensified due to the advancement of embryonic stem (ES) cell research. Numerous scientists and experts contend that stem cells derived from human blastocysts may be coaxed to form any kind of human cell or tissue for replacement and can possibly cure diseases that are the result of tissue degeneration, such as Parkinson's and Alzheimer's diseases. Supporters argue that federal funding for ES cell research is urgently needed in order to realize the full potential of ES cells. They insist that because blastocysts lack sentience, they cannot be categorized as live human beings. Therefore, federal funding of such research does not violate the existing law. In addition, supporters state that current ES experiments only involve the use of ES cell lines, cells grown in a culture, and not the actual blastocysts. On the other hand, detractors of ES cell research maintain that in order to create ES cell lines, blastocysts must be destroyed, an act they consider unethical. Furthermore, they argue that supporting human embryo experimentation affirms the utilitarian belief that human beings, without their consent, can justifiably be used to achieve the greater good of society.

On January 15, 1999, the U.S. Department of Health and Human Services (DHHS) made the controversial decision that federal funds may be used to support human ES cell research since the ES cells collected from embryos are not in themselves embryos. However, in August 2001, President George W. Bush changed the policy established by the DHHS, restricting the access of federal funds to ES research that will only use ES cell lines already in existence. Research that will harvest stem cells from blastocysts to create new cell lines is ineligible. In explaining his decision, Bush concluded that "the decision on life and death has already been made" for those blastocysts that have been destroyed to create the existing ES cell lines.

Bush's judgment regarding ES cell research has not dampened the controversy. The development of cloning technology in recent years has added to the debate. Numerous scientists want to clone embryos from which to harvest ES cells in order to explore the full capabilities of stem cell technology. For example, it is believed that cloning an embryo from a patient's cells will allow doctors to create tissue with which to treat that patient. This process could eliminate the problem of tissue rejection—a long-standing challenge in organ transplantation. Driven by the possibilities that human cloning may offer to ES cell technology, private biotechnological companies such as Advanced Cell Technology (ACT) are conducting human embryo cloning experiments without support from the federal government. According to their latest announcements, ACT successfully cloned human embryos in November 2001.

As of February 2002, Congress had yet to decide whether or not human cloning for any reason should be banned in the United States. In anticipation of new guidelines for human embryo experimentation, the authors in *At Issue: Human Embryo Experimentation* analyze and compare the possible benefits and costs of such research and debate its potential societal and ethical implications.

1

Embryonic Stem Cell Research Is Beneficial

National Institutes of Health

The National Institutes of Health (NIH), a branch of the U.S. Department of Health and Human Services, is a biomedical research center that seeks to discover new, effective medical treatments.

Embryonic stem (ES) cell research is vital to the advancement of medicine. ES cells are pluripotent—they can give rise to many human cells—and have many potential medical applications. For instance, isolating pluripotent cells can offer deeper insight into cell processes, cancer, and birth defects. Additionally, pluripotent stem cells have the far-reaching potential to treat diseases such as Parkinson's and heart disease, that are the result of cellular dysfunction. For example, the stem cells can provide a renewable source of cells and tissues for replacement. Although stem cells have been isolated from adult tissues, these cells have limited capabilities in comparison to stem cells derived from embryos.

This viewpoint presents background information on stem cells. It includes an explanation of what stem cells are; what pluripotent stem cells are; how pluripotent stem cells are derived; why pluripotent stem cells are important to science; why they hold such great promise for advances in health care; and what adult stem cells are.

Recent published reports on the isolation and successful culturing of the first human pluripotent stem cell lines have generated great excitement and have brought biomedical research to the edge of a new frontier. The development of these human pluripotent stem cell lines deserves close scientific examination, evaluation of the promise for new therapies and prevention strategies, and open discussion of the ethical issues.

In order to understand the importance of this discovery as well as the related scientific, medical, and ethical issues, it is absolutely essential to first clarify the terms and definitions.

Excerpted from "Stem Cells: A Primer," by the National Institutes of Health, www.nih.gov, May 2000.

What is a stem cell?

Stem cells have the ability to divide for indefinite periods in culture and to give rise to specialized cells. They are best described in the context of normal human development. Human development begins when a sperm fertilizes an egg and creates a single cell that has the potential to form an entire organism. This fertilized egg is totipotent, meaning that its potential is total. In the first hours after fertilization, this cell divides into identical totipotent cells. This means that either one of these cells, if placed into a woman's uterus, has the potential to develop into a fetus. In fact, identical twins develop when two totipotent cells separate and develop into two individual, genetically identical human beings. Approximately four days after fertilization and after several cycles of cell division, these totipotent cells begin to specialize, forming a hollow sphere of cells, called a blastocyst. The blastocyst has an outer layer of cells and inside the hollow sphere, there is a cluster of cells called the inner cell mass.

The outer layer of cells will go on to form the placenta and other supporting tissues needed for fetal development in the uterus. The inner cell mass cells will go on to form virtually all of the tissues of the human body. Although the inner cell mass cells can form virtually every type of cell found in the human body, they cannot form an organism because they are unable to give rise to the placenta and supporting tissues necessary for development in the human uterus. These inner cell mass cells are pluripotent—they can give rise to many types of cells but not all types of cells necessary for fetal development. Because their potential is not total, they are not totipotent and they are not embryos. In fact, if an inner cell mass cell were placed into a woman's uterus, it would not develop into a fetus.

The pluripotent stem cells undergo further specialization into stem cells that are committed to give rise to cells that have a particular function. Examples of this include blood stem cells which give rise to red blood cells, white blood cells and platelets; and skin stem cells that give rise to the various types of skin cells. These more specialized stem cells are called multipotent.

While stem cells are extraordinarily important in early human development, multipotent stem cells are also found in children and adults. For example, consider one of the best understood stem cells, the blood stem cell. Blood stem cells reside in the bone marrow of every child and adult, and in fact, they can be found in very small numbers circulating in the blood stream. Blood stem cells perform the critical role of continually replenishing our supply of blood cells—red blood cells, white blood cells, and platelets— throughout life. A person cannot survive without blood stem cells.

How are pluripotent stem cells derived?

At present, human pluripotent cell lines have been developed from two sources[1] with methods previously developed in work with animal models.

(1) In the work done by Dr. James Thomson, pluripotent stem cells were isolated directly from the inner cell mass of human embryos at the blastocyst stage. Dr. Thomson received embryos from IVF (In Vitro Fertilization) clinics—these embryos were in excess of the clinical need for infertility treatment. The embryos were made for purposes of reproduction,

not research. Informed consent was obtained from the donor couples. Dr. Thomson isolated the inner cell mass and cultured these cells producing a pluripotent stem cell line.

(2) In contrast, Dr. John Gearhart isolated pluripotent stem cells from fetal tissue obtained from terminated pregnancies. Informed consent was obtained from the donors after they had independently made the decision to terminate their pregnancy. Dr. Gearhart took cells from the region of the fetus that was destined to develop into the testes or the ovaries. Although the cells developed in Dr. Gearhart's lab and Dr. Thomson's lab were derived from different sources, they appear to be very similar.

Pluripotent stem cells could help us to understand the complex events that occur during human development.

The use of somatic cell nuclear transfer (SCNT) may be another way that pluripotent stem cells could be isolated. In studies with animals using SCNT, researchers take a normal animal egg cell and remove the nucleus (cell structure containing the chromosomes). The material left behind in the egg cell contains nutrients and other energy-producing materials that are essential for embryo development. Then, using carefully worked out laboratory conditions, a somatic cell—any cell other than an egg or a sperm cell—is placed next to the egg from which the nucleus had been removed, and the two are fused. The resulting fused cell, and its immediate descendants, are believed to have the full potential to develop into an entire animal, and hence are totipotent. These totipotent cells will soon form a blastocyst. Cells from the inner cell mass of this blastocyst could, in theory, be used to develop pluripotent stem cell lines. Indeed, any method by which a human blastocyst is formed could potentially serve as a source of human pluripotent stem cells.

Potential applications of pluripotent stem cells

There are several important reasons why the isolation of human pluripotent stem cells is important to science and to advances in health care. At the most fundamental level, pluripotent stem cells could help us to understand the complex events that occur during human development. A primary goal of this work would be the identification of the factors involved in the cellular decision-making process that results in cell specialization. We know that turning genes on and off is central to this process, but we do not know much about these "decision-making" genes or what turns them on or off. Some of our most serious medical conditions, such as cancer and birth defects, are due to abnormal cell specialization and cell division. A better understanding of normal cell processes will allow us to further delineate the fundamental errors that cause these often deadly illnesses.

Human pluripotent stem cell research could also dramatically change the way we develop drugs and test them for safety. For example, new medications could be initially tested using human cell lines. Cell lines are currently used in this way (for example cancer cells). Pluripotent stem cells would allow testing in more cell types. This would not replace testing in whole animals and testing in human beings, but it would streamline the process of drug development. Only the drugs that are both safe and appear to have a beneficial effect in cell line testing would graduate to further testing in laboratory animals and human subjects.

Perhaps the most far-reaching potential application of human pluripotent stem cells is the generation of cells and tissue that could be used for so-called "cell therapies." Many diseases and disorders result from disruption of cellular function or destruction of tissues of the body. Today, donated organs and tissues are often used to replace ailing or destroyed tissue. Unfortunately, the number of people suffering from these disorders far outstrips the number of organs available for transplantation. Pluripotent stem cells, stimulated to develop into specialized cells, offer the possibility of a renewable source of replacement cells and tissue to treat a myriad of diseases, conditions, and disabilities including Parkinson's and Alzheimer's diseases, spinal cord injury, stroke, burns, heart disease, diabetes, osteoarthritis and rheumatoid arthritis. There is almost no realm of medicine that might not be touched by this innovation. Some details of two of these examples follow.

- Transplant of healthy heart muscle cells could provide new hope for patients with chronic heart disease whose hearts can no longer pump adequately. The hope is to develop heart muscle cells from human pluripotent stem cells and transplant them into the failing heart muscle in order to augment the function of the failing heart. Preliminary work in mice and other animals has demonstrated that healthy heart muscle cells transplanted into the heart successfully repopulate the heart tissue and work together with the host cells. These experiments show that this type of transplantation is feasible.
- In the many individuals who suffer from Type I diabetes, the production of insulin by specialized pancreatic cells, called islet cells, is disrupted. There is evidence that transplantation of either the entire pancreas or isolated islet cells could mitigate the need for insulin injections. Islet cell lines derived from human pluripotent stem cells could be used for diabetes research and, ultimately, for transplantation.

Human pluripotent stem cell research could also dramatically change the way we develop drugs and test them for safety.

While this research shows extraordinary promise, there is much to be done before we can realize these innovations. Technological challenges remain before these discoveries can be incorporated into clinical practice. These challenges, though significant, are not insurmountable.

First, we must do the basic research to understand the cellular events that lead to cell specialization in the human, so that we can direct these pluripotent stem cells to become the type(s) of tissue needed for transplantation.

Second, before we can use these cells for transplantation, we must overcome the well-known problem of immune rejection. Because human pluripotent stem cells derived from embryos or fetal tissue would be genetically different from the recipient, future research would need to focus on modifying human pluripotent stem cells to minimize tissue incompatibility or to create tissue banks with the most common tissue-type profiles.

The use of somatic cell nuclear transfer (SCNT) would be another way to overcome the problem of tissue incompatibility for some patients. For example, consider a person with progressive heart failure. Using SCNT, the nucleus of virtually any somatic cell from that patient could be fused with a donor egg cell from which the nucleus had been removed. With proper stimulation the cell would develop into a blastocyst: cells from the inner cell mass could be taken to create a culture of pluripotent cells. These cells could then be stimulated to develop into heart muscle cells. Because the vast majority of genetic information is contained in the nucleus, these cells would be essentially identical genetically to the person with the failing heart. When these heart muscle cells were transplanted back into the patient, there would likely be no rejection and no need to expose the patient to immune-suppressing drugs, which can have toxic effects.

Adult stem cells

As noted earlier, multipotent stem cells can be found in some types of adult tissue. In fact, stem cells are needed to replenish the supply cells in our body that normally wear out. An example, which was mentioned previously, is the blood stem cell.

Multipotent stem cells have not been found for all types of adult tissue, but discoveries in this area of research are increasing. For example, until recently, it was thought that stem cells were not present in the adult nervous system, but, in recent years, neuronal stem cells have been isolated from the rat and mouse nervous systems. The experience in humans is more limited. In humans, neuronal stem cells have been isolated from fetal tissue and a kind of cell that may be a neuronal stem cell has been isolated from adult brain tissue that was surgically removed for the treatment of epilepsy.

Pluripotent stem cells . . . offer the possibility of a renewable source of replacement cells and tissue to treat a myriad of diseases.

Do adult stem cells have the same potential as pluripotent stem cells?

Until recently, there was little evidence in mammals that multipotent cells such as blood stem cells could change course and produce skin cells, liver cells or any cell other than a blood stem cell or a specific type of blood cell; however, research in animals is leading scientists to question this view.

In animals, it has been shown that some adult stem cells previously thought to be committed to the development of one line of specialized cells are able to develop into other types of specialized cells. For example, recent experiments in mice suggest that when neural stem cells were placed into the bone marrow, they appeared to produce a variety of blood cell types. In addition, studies with rats have indicated that stem cells found in the bone marrow were able to produce liver cells. These exciting findings suggest that even after a stem cell has begun to specialize, the stem cell may, under certain conditions, be more flexible than first thought. At this time, demonstration of the flexibility of adult stem cells has been only observed in animals and limited to a few tissue types.

Why not just pursue research with adult stem cells?

Research on human adult stem cells suggests that these multipotent cells have great potential for use in both research and in the development of cell therapies. For example, there would be many advantages to using adult stem cells for transplantation. If we could isolate the adult stem cells from a patient, coax them to divide and direct their specialization and then transplant them back into the patient, it is unlikely that such cells would be rejected. The use of adult stem cells for such cell therapies would certainly reduce or even avoid the practice of using stem cells that were derived from human embryos or human fetal tissue, sources that trouble many people on ethical grounds.

While adult stem cells hold real promise, there are some significant limitations to what we may or may not be able to accomplish with them.

While adult stem cells hold real promise, there are some significant limitations to what we may or may not be able to accomplish with them. First of all, stem cells from adults have not been isolated for all tissues of the body. Although many different kinds of multipotent stem cells have been identified, adult stem cells for all cell and tissue types have not yet been found in the adult human. For example, we have not located adult cardiac stem cells or adult pancreatic islet stem cells in humans.

Secondly, adult stem cells are often present in only minute quantities, are difficult to isolate and purify, and their numbers may decrease with age. For example, brain cells from adults that may be neuronal stem cells have only been obtained by removing a portion of the brain of epileptics, not a trivial procedure.

Any attempt to use stem cells from a patient's own body for treatment would require that stem cells would first have to be isolated from the patient and then grown in culture in sufficient numbers to obtain adequate quantities for treatment. For some acute disorders, there may not be enough time to grow enough cells to use for treatment. In other disorders, caused by a genetic defect, the genetic error would likely be present in the patient's stem cells. Cells from such a patient may not be appropriate for transplantation. There is evidence that stem cells from adults may not have the same capacity to proliferate as younger cells do. In addition, adult stem cells may contain more DNA abnormalities, caused by exposure to daily living, including sunlight, toxins, and by expected errors made in DNA replication during the course of a lifetime. These potential weaknesses could limit the usefulness of adult stem cells.

Research on the early stages of cell specialization may not be possible with adult stem cells since they appear to be farther along the specialization pathway than pluripotent stem cells. In addition, one adult stem cell line may be able to form several, perhaps 3 or 4, tissue types, but there is no clear evidence that stem cells from adults, human or animal, are pluripotent. In fact, there is no evidence that adult stem cells have the broad potential characteristic of pluripotent stem cells. In order to determine the very best source of many of the specialized cells and tissues of the body for new treatments and even cures, it will be vitally important to study the developmental potential of adult stem cells and compare it to that of pluripotent stem cells.

The enormous promise of stem cells

Given the enormous promise of stem cells to the development of new therapies for the most devastating diseases, it is important to simultaneously pursue all lines of research. Science and scientists need to search for the very best sources of these cells. When they are identified, regardless of their sources, researchers will use them to pursue the development of new cell therapies.

The development of stem cell lines, both pluripotent and multipotent, that may produce many tissues of the human body is an important scientific breakthrough. It is not too unrealistic to say that this research has the potential to revolutionize the practice of medicine and improve the quality and length of life.

Note

1. Michael Shamblott, *et al*, Derivation of pluripotent stem cells from cultured human primordial germ cells. *PNAS*, 95: 13726–13731, Nov. 1998.

   James Thomson, *et al*, Embryonic stem cell lines derived from human blastocysts. *Science*, 282: 1145–1147, Nov. 6, 1998.

2

Human Embryo Experimentation Can Be Morally Justifiable

Michael J. Meyer and Lawrence J. Nelson

Michael J. Meyer is an associate professor and department chair of philosophy at Santa Clara University in California. Lawrence J. Nelson is a lecturer of philosophy at Santa Clara University and has served as a bioethics consultant to the National Institutes of Health.

The potentially groundbreaking field of embryonic stem cell research relies upon the use and destruction of human embryos in the earliest stages of development. Opponents of such research argue that human embryos deserve the moral respect of human beings and should not be experimented upon. However, the destruction of human embryos for justifiable scientific experimentation does not necessarily undermine their moral status. For example, the present-day use of human cadavers in medical research demonstrates how objects destroyed during scientific experimentation can be treated with respect. Researchers dissect human cadavers respectfully, in an effort to expand scientific knowledge of the human body.

How can one have moral respect for something that one intentionally destroys? This perplexing question is pointedly raised by several commentators on the ethics of human stem cell and embryo research when they claim that extracorporeal embryos at one and the same time merit "profound respect,"[1] "respect . . . for [their] special character,"[2] or "special respect,"[3] and yet remain suitable for use in scientific research that results in their destruction. Daniel Callahan [senior fellow at the Harvard Medical School], among others, has puzzled about how the extracorporeal embryo can be both "entitled to profound respect" and also sacrificed "in deference to the requirements of research."[4] The puzzle for Callahan, and for us here, is how we can, without a tragic disingenuousness, accede to "the killing of something for which [we] claim to have a profound re-

From "Respecting What We Destroy: Reflections on Human Embryo Research," by Michael J. Meyer and Lawrence J. Nelson, *Hastings Center Report*, January/February 2001. Copyright © 2001 by The Hastings Center. Reprinted with permission.

spect." The puzzle raises two questions: Does not having an attitude of respect for something rule out its ultimate destruction? Second, even if this is not so, is not the research use and destruction of embryos "more honestly done by simply stripping [these] embryos of any value at all?"

Our answer to both questions is no. What respect requires can be an alternative both to a prohibition on destruction and to a moral license to kill. We will argue that a genuine moral respect for embryos can be joined—without incongruity but not without careful attention to how that respect is displayed—with their use and destruction in legitimate research. This is of course not meant to be a description of the moral attitudes that people typically have about embryos. Our conclusion is rather an evocation of a moral ideal especially worthy of recognition at a time when research using human embryos is likely to escalate.[5]

Before taking up the moral compatibility between respecting something and destroying it, we first provide a brief account of moral status in general and then address the particular moral status of embryos. The moral status of an entity must be clarified before the moral permissibility of its intentional destruction can be ascertained. It is to the question of moral status, then, that we turn first.

Moral status and respect

There are nonmoral uses of the idea of respect—like the respect one might have for a heavyweight champion's left hook or a scholar's opinion. An agent evinces *moral* respect, however, when he or she sincerely considers and actually treats an entity as worthy of some degree of deference, reverence, or regard. Plainly, this kind of respect is dependent on a reckoning of the entity's moral status. An entity toward which moral agents have direct obligations, or whose needs, interests, or well-being require protection, for example, will also command respect.[6] Moral agents clearly have a rather high moral status, and they correspondingly deserve very significant moral respect.

However, moral respect should not be collapsed into an account of respect for moral agents or their characteristics. Humans who are not agents or not yet agents, sentient creatures, other living things, species, and biotic communities are all sometimes said to have moral status and deserve moral respect. Of course, if such widely varying kinds of entities are accorded moral status, the notions of moral status and respect must admit of degrees.[7] Plainly, too, people differ in what they assign status and accord respect to. Nonetheless, any attribution of moral status, however weak, must be taken seriously by others.

We employ the method of ascertaining moral status recently elaborated by [philosophy professor] Mary Anne Warren, who has argued convincingly that no one criterion can determine moral status. In fact, for Warren, a judgment about an entity's moral status involves seven different principles, which include both intrinsic and relational properties of the entity in question. In abbreviated form, Warren's seven principles are: (1) *respect for life:* living organisms may not be killed or harmed without good reasons; (2) *anti-cruelty:* sentient beings ought not to be killed or subjected to pain unless there is no other way of furthering goals that are both consistent with the other principles and important to entities that have higher moral status than can be based on sentience alone; (3) *agent's rights:* moral agents have full and equal moral rights, including rights to life and liberty; (4) *human rights:* within the limits of their capacities, human beings capable of sentience but not moral agency have the same moral rights as moral agents; (5) *ecological importance:* ecologically important entities (living and nonliving) may have a stronger moral status than they would independent of their relationship to the ecosystem; (6) *interspecific communities:* animals that are part of a human community may have stronger moral status than they would standing alone; (7) *transitivity of respect:* within the limits of the above principles and to the extent that is reasonable, moral agents should respect one another's attributions of moral status.[8]

Transitivity of respect

Our account of moral respect will draw on Warren's work. In this account, moral agents have the highest moral status and possess full and equal basic moral rights. An individual who displays only minimal consciousness has the same basic moral rights and status as an agent, even though he lacks those rights his diminished capacities render irrelevant.[9] Nonhuman but sentient creatures possess a moral status that is significant but typically less than that of humans. Other, nonsentient living entities have even lower status but still merit some, even if in most cases quite minimal, moral respect.

A genuine moral respect for embryos can be joined . . . with their use and destruction in legitimate research.

If Warren's account is right, human embryos have a weak moral status and deserve a weak but genuine moral respect. The moral status of embryos does not, contrary to the suggestion of some, rest exclusively on their being the result of reproductive activity.[10] Rather, the human embryo has a claim to some moral status both in virtue of being alive and in virtue of Warren's rule of the "transitivity of respect." Although frozen embryos are in a state of suspended animation, they are still living entities, and purely gratuitous harm to or destruction of a living thing is, many would say, clearly morally problematic. When a living thing is harmed or destroyed there must be some reasonable justification for doing so. Thus while the claim that life itself is worthy of moral respect is surely controversial, it is hardly unusual, and indeed seems rather plausible if moral respect is held to admit of different levels.

The moral status of embryos also turns on the fact that, in addition to being alive, they are valued, in some cases very highly, by many people. The value ascribed to an embryo covers a wide range, of course; it is sometimes essentially given the full worth and status of a moral agent,[11] sometimes a very high status but not at every stage the equal of a moral agent,[12] and sometimes only very modest moral status. Some hold that an extracorporeal human embryo naturally engenders a sense of wonder, or that it is a thing of beauty.[13] What gives rise to these reactions provides a reason to hold that the extracorporeal embryo has some modest moral status. One might, for instance, have a sense of wonder about embryos because of the simple realization that an embryo is, in some rough sense, "the stuff of life." Its beauty alone is also a distinct reason to accord it some moral status.

The transitivity principle does not depend on a defense of any particular view an agent might hold about the embryo's moral status. The whole point of the transitivity principle is that the actual valuations of other agents merit respect even when one does not share their valuations. According some respect to the value judgments of others does not entail that one shares those value judgments, even less that one has abandoned one's own values, but simply that one has some respect for the individuals who *do* have those values. Stones may be uninteresting to us, but we nonetheless should recognize some obligation to protect rock formations that are sacred to others, as Uluru is for Australian aboriginals or Shiprock for the Navajo. Respect for the moral agency of others requires us to not dismiss their views lightly. Demonstrating this respect is one aspect of showing respect for one's fellow agents. To suggest instead that moral views that depart from one's own should be dismissed is not only to court dogmatism, but also to fail to establish reasonable and principled common ground with those who have divergent views of complex moral problems.[14]

Neither an agent nor an entity

Surely, then, there is good reason to say that the extracorporeal embryo has some moral status and is worthy of some moral respect. More specifically, our interpretation of Warren's account leads us to conclude that its status is weak or modest. The only intrinsic property that provides a reason to grant it moral status is its being alive. The embryo is neither an agent, a human being capable of sentience but not agency, a nonhuman sentient creature, nor an entity of ecological significance. Nor is an embryo a person, or an early stage of a person, in the typical understandings, both metaphysical and moral, of the muddled term "person."[15] One oft-noted reason it isn't is that an embryo prior to the formation of the "primitive streak" (which usually appears around fourteen days of development) is not clearly even an *individual*, as it can still be divided into twins. Personhood is usually taken to imply individuality.[16] Another reason is that, if an embryo is maintained outside a woman's body and those who provided the gametes for it have not decided to permit its development in a womb, it is not effectively a stage in the early development of a person. Put differently, an extracorporeal embryo—whether used in research, discarded, or kept frozen—is simply not a precursor to any ongoing personal narrative. An embryo properly starts on that trajectory only when the gamete sources intentionally have it placed in a womb.

We recognize that reasonable people will continue to disagree about the moral status of embryos. Indeed, the very recent appearance of the extracorporeal embryo (it did not exist before the 1970s) provides reason to think that disagreement about its moral status is more than understandable. Our goal, however, is not to provide a knock-down argument about the moral status of the embryo, but to show how one systematic, reasonable view on moral status in general can be used to defend the moral propriety of destroying embryos that truly deserve respect. For this defense to succeed, it is necessary that the status of the embryo be assessed as only modest or weak.

Nevertheless, possession of even weak *moral* status supports the claim that embryos deserve "special" respect. Something's entitlement to even weak moral status requires that there be sincere moral deliberation about its treatment. Those who doubt the force of this point underestimate the importance of the line between the moral and nonmoral. The very presence of moral status demands sincere and genuine reflection on questions like: What level of respectful treatment do I owe this entity? What would a morally admirable person do to this entity, and what should I in good conscience refuse to do to it? In contrast, all such questions are simply beside the point for entities without moral status.

The moral status of embryos does not, contrary to the suggestion of some, rest exclusively on their being the result of reproductive activity.

When we are considering an entity that has any moral status, destruction, harm, or any other disrespectful treatment cannot be justified by our self-interest alone. Our account of the moral status of human embryos entails that they deserve some respect in all contexts, even when they are destroyed for good reason. Whenever the forces of moral deliberation are called into play on behalf of an entity having even weak moral status, reasonable and conscientious persons clearly are required to give due regard to the entity in question as well as to the manner in which their actions regarding it affect their own moral character.

Respecting while destroying

The moral respect an agent has for something or someone is demonstrated in two fundamental ways: in what the agent does or refuses to do with the object of respect, and in the attitudes the agent adopts in relation to that which he or she respects. Behavior must be consistent with attitude; someone cannot legitimately claim he or she holds a respectful attitude about something while his or her behavior clearly manifests indifference, disregard, or contempt. Morally respectful behavior can assume a variety of forms: addressing the respected entity in a certain manner, protecting and preserving it from destruction or degradation, thinking of it or talking about it in terms that accurately reflect its value, and encouraging or requiring others to behave respectfully. The precise forms of respectful behavior adopted by an agent should also be congruent with the degree of respect owed to the particular object in question. To solve the puzzle of how we can show respect for what we destroy, we must recognize the moral weight of both the sincerely respectful attitude of the destroying agent toward the destroyed object, as well as the purposefully adopted behavioral manifestations of this attitude.

Sometimes people destroy something *because* they respect it, as when a sacred artifact is destroyed to prevent its being treated in a profane way. In contrast, embryos are destroyed in the course of research *in spite of* the respect they deserve. Destroying an object in spite of the respect it is owed raises the tension we seek to resolve. To illustrate how the tension might be resolved, we offer some actual examples of people who have destroyed what they truly respect.

An extracorporeal embryo—whether used in research, discarded, or kept frozen—is simply not a precursor to any ongoing personal narrative.

A variety of Native American hunting cultures manifested a "very close relationship between man and game animals" that was grounded in their religious beliefs as well as in the ritual attitudes they maintained and practices they observed with respect to these animals.[17] For these peoples, all living beings are "associated with and related to one another socially and sociably," as humans are to each other. They did not see animals as objects, but as "fellows with whom the individual or band may have a more or less advantageous relationship."[18] These Native Americans also believed supernatural masters or owners of the game animals existed who cared about the way the animals were treated and would punish hunters who kill excessively or show other disrespectful behavior toward the animals.[19]

The Cree and Micmac cultures, to pick two examples, expressed their respect for the animals they destroyed in a wide variety of ways. Some addressed the animal by a familial name such as "Grandmother" or "Cousin" or by an honorary title like "Chief's Son" or "Four-Legged Human."[20] They demonstrated respect or esteem by killing animals only with aboriginal weapons and by making a conciliatory speech to the animal, either before or after killing it (and sometimes both), "by which the hunter sincerely apologizes for the necessity of his act."[21] They maintained a reverent atmosphere while eating a bear and carefully avoided wasting any of it—even avoiding spilling into the fire any soup made from the animal.[22] Finally, they showed respect for the animal's remains by never throwing its bones into the fire or giving them to the dogs, and sometimes they went so far as to bury the animal's bones in anatomical order.[23]

Memorials for the aborted

The Japanese practice of *mizuko kuyo* can be understood as another demonstration of respect for what is destroyed, in this case the aborted human fetus. *Mizuko kuyo* includes a variety of spiritual rituals initiated primarily by women as memorial services for their aborted fetuses. These rituals include saying prayers, making floral offerings, burning incense, lighting candies, creating wooden plaques called *ema* that carry prayers for, and messages to, the fetuses (such as "please sleep peacefully" or "please forgive me"), and making reverential bows to the *mizuko jizo*, a statuary image that represents the soul of the deceased fetus and the deity that cares for departed children. One commentator has noted that although the content of the ritual varies widely, they all aim "uniformly to comfort and honor" the spirits of the aborted fetuses.[24] In addition, some of those who perform *mizuko kuyo* rituals do so partly because they wish to make a public demonstration that they acted responsibly. Others have the "desire to register publicly their belief that they did not abort unfeelingly or callously." Older women especially do not perform the ritual "in shame or fear" so much as to "give public recognition to an act that for them was both sorrowful and unavoidable."

Naomi Wolf has argued that the struggle for abortion rights should be placed within a moral framework that urges all discussions about "destroy[ing] a manifestation of life" be characterized by "grief and respect."[25] For those who believe that "abortion is killing and yet [are] still prochoice," Wolf suggests that they engage in "acts of redemption, or what the Jewish mystical tradition calls *tikkun*, or 'mending.'" She provides several examples of such acts, one of which is to suggest that mothers or fathers who were involved in an abortion can "remember the aborted child every time [they are] tempted to be less than loving—and give renewed love to [a] living child." Such acts of *tikkun*, as well as the practice of *mizuko kuyo*, are manifestations of genuine respect for the aborted fetus, even if that respect was by itself not enough to lead a woman to forgo the abortion.

Human cadavers

The contemporary treatment of human cadavers in medical schools provides another example of treating with respect that which is destroyed. All known societies have had customs delineating the proper treatment of the bodies of the dead.[26] These customs mostly are characterized by the value and respect paid to the bodies and the consequent revulsion experienced by encountering desecration of corpses or other acts of disrespect. Antigone defied at great risk her king's order to leave her brother's body unburied, and therefore in disgrace, in order to obey what she saw as her moral duty to bury him with respect. Dissection of human cadavers for educational or scientific purposes was widely condemned for hundreds of years, although the need for dissection led physicians and others to rob graves or to use bodies unclaimed by relatives. Dissection was so disfavored in the United States that one state legally banned it until 1887, and another made it a "punishment" for having been killed while dueling.[27]

Respect for human cadavers is ethically grounded in the very close identification of persons and their bodies and in the association of the human form with living human beings themselves. "[W]hile the body retains a recognizable form, even in death, it commands the respect of identity," notes William May. "No longer a human presence, it still reminds us of the presence that once was utterly inseparable from it."[28] In addition, cadavers are especially honored by those who had personal relationships with the persons while alive, and others are bound by the transitivity principle to respect both the cadaver and those who hold it in special regard. The respect that is owed to cadavers is reflected in the honorific rituals of institutions which make scientific and educational use of cadavers:

While [the memorial services held prior to burial or crema-
tion of dissected remains] take a variety of forms, their aim
is to honor those who have donated their bodies to an
anatomy department for the purposes of teaching and research. This serves as a formal and public demonstration of
anatomy departments' appreciation for such bequests.
Whether secular or ecumenical, such services bring together
the altruism of the donors, the gratitude of the students and
faculty, and the memories of close relatives and friends.[29]

In addition, students and researchers should, and do, show respect
for cadavers during their use and destruction of them.

Conscientious treatment

The conscientious treatment shown to dissected cadavers clearly displays
the respect that they are widely thought to be owed. Likewise the re-
demptive acts of *tikkun* and the rituals of *mizuko kuya* deserve to be understood in light of the recognition that the persons who engage in them
are showing a special respect for what they have intentionally destroyed.
And the Native American rituals have meaning only given the understanding that the hunter who has destroyed the animals did have some
deep and genuine respect for them.

Now it is not our present point to defend either these specific practices or the complex set of moral evaluations out of which they arise. Instead, we want first to make the more limited point that there is no inherent conceptual contradiction or severe moral dilemma involved in the
general idea of showing respect for what one destroys. The examples afford a few authentic instances of the general practice of respecting what
one destroys.

Second, although we do not wish to argue for the precise form of respectful, compensatory acknowledgment for either animals, fetuses, cadavers, or even embryos, the examples provide a rough idea of some of
the typical features of respecting what one destroys. They suggest that respecting what one destroys should include an attitude of regret, and some
sense of loss, conjoined with a display of that respect. Respecting what is
destroyed should include an attitude of regret and loss because the thing
one has intentionally destroyed does in fact have moral value. Even the
gains reaped through its destruction do not preclude honest and open acknowledgment of the regret and loss one should feel about it.

Gamete sources, respect, and the
disposition of extracorporeal embryos

The persons most humanly and morally connected to any particular extracorporeal embryo are the individual women and men from whom the
gametes came. These persons have a special connection to any embryo
they create for two reasons. First, as the embryo is wholly constituted by
the gametes that were part of, indeed a genetic representation of, the persons from whom they came, these gamete sources are uniquely connected to the embryo biologically and ontologically. Without these gametes the particular embryo in question simply would not exist.

Second, the gamete sources also have a genuine moral connection to their embryos. This may be grounded in either a particular interest they might take in those of their embryos not designated for reproductive uses, or a potentially profound interest they might take in an embryo that is designated for reproduction. Most persons care deeply if their gametes are used, by themselves or others, to create a child, and being a genetic parent can understandably be linked in deep ways to an individual's sense of identity and of the meaning of life. In a clearly different but still meaningful way, gamete sources might well care about how their embryo is used by others for research purposes. They might believe, for example, that the embryo has independent moral value. They might also feel that it simply belongs to him or her and that no one else should be using it. Furthermore, it is implausible that someone other than a gamete source would have a more significant moral connection to a particular embryo.

As a direct result of the special biological, ontological, and moral connection between embryos and the persons whose gametes are used to create them, the latter should jointly exercise the right of exclusive control over the disposition of those embryos, whether they be used immediately or later for personal reproductive use, donated to others for reproductive purposes, donated to research, or just discarded. This deep interest in the valuation of and control over an embryo is closely related to an individual's interest in and right to make intimate, personal decisions. This interest should prevail over conflicting views others may have of the embryo's moral value or of what may be done with it. Therefore, the voluntary, informed consent of the gamete sources is morally required for any disposition of their embryos, and others ought to respect the terms and conditions the gamete sources place on this disposition.

The gamete sources may confer on their own embryos a moral status higher than the minimum status we argued for earlier in this paper. If they do, they might refuse either to donate their embryos for research or to destroy any of them and might try instead to bring all of them eventually to birth. Treating their embryos this way violates none of the moral duties they owe to others. Given their prerogative to grant their own embryos more than minimal moral status, the gamete sources are not morally obliged to permit their embryos to be used by someone else for reproduction or research. Put differently, no one should be morally or legally[30] compelled either to become a genetic parent through use of his or her embryos or to donate one's own embryo for any legitimate or worthy use by another. If the case in favor of giving all embryos higher moral status and more respectful treatment could be made convincingly to others, then many more, maybe even most, gamete sources would refuse to donate embryos to research. Still, no moral wrong would thereby be done to researchers or to humankind, even though a potential good would be delayed or forgone.

Baseline requirements

While the gamete sources may stipulate special restrictions on how an embryo is to be treated, there are also some general, base-line requirements for the treatment of an embryo. No moral agent can properly deem an extracorporeal embryo—whether someone else's or hers—morally worthless. Although the *disposition* of extracorporeal embryos "belongs" to the gamete sources who created them, the embryos are not like simple proprietary objects that can be regarded by their owners as valueless. As we argued above embryos have genuine, if modest, moral status and deserve genuine respect both because they are alive and because they are regarded by others as morally valuable.

If embryos are acknowledged to have only a weak moral status, nothing wrong is done to any embryo if the gamete sources voluntarily donate them, with a respectful acknowledgment of their moral status, for use in legitimate research—research, that is, that utilizes sound scientific methodology and design and possesses the reasonable promise of generating significant knowledge, whether theoretical or practical in nature.[31] While significance is surely a matter of degree, significant knowledge is at least not trivial. It would not, for instance, be clearly unnecessary repetition of established results. In addition, legitimate research neither involves morally objectionable acts nor is predominantly intended to generate publicity, economic value, or achieve some other end at the direct expense of developing generalizable knowledge.

Our account of the moral status of human embryos entails that they deserve some respect in all contexts, even when they are destroyed.

Donating embryos for such research, even though it involves their destruction, can be consistent with genuine respect for them, because of their weak moral status. Such use and destruction would be by itself disrespectful if it were moral agents who were used in research, but for embryos destruction is not inherently unacceptable, *provided* both that the gamete sources consent to this use and that the extracorporeal embryo receives respectful treatment, proportional to its moral status. A variety of attitudes and practices can demonstrate respectful acknowledgment of the moral status of extracorporeal embryos. In the context of research with embryos, both gamete sources and researchers are the parties most immediately obligated to make such respectful acknowledgment. The duties of the two might also be linked in the following way: examples of how researchers might show respect, or avoid showing disrespect, can be understood as cases of what gamete sources could request, or require, from the researchers to whom they donate their extracorporeal embryos.

Restrictions on the treatment of embryos

Examples of restrictions on the treatment of embryos that would show respect for them (which are independent of justifications for their destruction) would include the following: (1) human extracorporeal embryos should be used in research only if the research goals cannot be obtained with other methods;[32] (2) the use of extracorporeal embryos more than fourteen days old should be avoided or diminished, since this point is regarded by some as the morally significant onset of embryonic individuation;[33] (3) researchers should avoid considering extracorporeal embryos as property and in particular should avoid buying and selling them; (4) researchers should recognize that the destruction of extracorporeal embryos provides a reason for them to have and demonstrate some sense of regret or loss. Further, handling extracorporeal embryos with respect in the lab should never be an empty or insincere gesture but might include both acquiring only the minimum number of embryos required to achieve the research goals and disposing of the remains of used embryos in a way respectful of their status (for example, the remains might be treated as if they were corpses and be buried or cremated).

While the embryo's moral status need not prevent us from killing it, it should nevertheless have some practical deterrent effect against killing it.

Thus while the embryo's moral status need not prevent us from killing it, it should nevertheless have some practical deterrent effect against killing it, since it requires that the destruction be for justifiable reasons, and that the destruction and eventual disposal in some way reflect the seriousness of the event. In our view no one ought to kill extracorporeal embryos for trivial reasons or in ways that would in fact fail to show respect for them. There is, in general, no reason to suppose that *any* level of moral status and respect should have a practical deterrent effect against *every* form of killing—even moral agents may be killed in self-defense. In short, the level of moral status and respect due to any particular entity will establish the level of justification required to render killing that entity permissible.

We leave open for further specification precisely what displays of respect are appropriate for embryos, but there must be some such displays or the accompanying use of extracorporeal embryos will be unethical.

Questions

Our attempt to show how we can reasonably combine genuine moral respect for extracorporeal embryos with their intentional destruction leaves a number of related issues deliberately untouched. These include: (1) the relationship between the moral status of the extracorporeal embryo and its legal status, and whether the law ought to enforce certain restrictions that would reflect respectful treatment (for example, banning commercial trade in embryos); (2) a set of further moral considerations, such as how the practices involved in respecting what one destroys help deepen habits of moral imagination and other subtleties of moral character; (3) whether some proponents of research distort its moral and practical value in order to justify the use of embryos; (4) what to do, morally or legally, if the gamete sources disagree on the disposition of their extracorporeal embryos; and (5) whether the intentional creation of embryos exclusively for research purposes can be morally justified.

We have sought to parry Callahan's suggestion that the use and destruction of human embryos is best justified "by simply stripping embryos of any value at all." Instead we have argued that given the minimal but real moral respect owed to an embryo, there can be, and ought to be, some display of respect whenever they are used, but that the destruction of an embryo need not display disrespect for it. Moreover, while the display of such respect could range widely in form and content, ignoring this display is in all likelihood a sign of a hardening of the heart that need not be part of our scientific progress.

References

1. Report of the HEW Ethics Advisory Board, *Research Involving In Vitro Fertilization and Embryo Transfer* (Washington, D.C.: U.S. Department of Health, Education, and Welfare, 4 May 1979), p. 101.

2. Human Embryo Research Panel of the National Institutes of Health, *Final Report of the Human Embryo Research Panel of the National Institutes of Health* (Bethesda, Md.: U.S. National Institutes of Health, 27 September 1994), p. 3.

3. John Robertson, "Symbolic Issues in Embryo Research," *Hastings Center Report* 25, no. 1 (1995), p. 37.

4. Daniel Callahan, "The Puzzle of Profound Respect," *Hastings Center Report* 25, no. 1 (1995), pp. 39–40.

5. Department of Health and Human Services, "National Institutes of Health Guidelines for Research Using Human Pluripotent Stem Cells," *Federal Register* 65, no. 166, 25 August 2000, pp. 51976–81.

6. Mary Anne Warren, *Moral Status: Obligations to Persons and Other Living Things* (Oxford: Oxford University Press, 1997), p. 3.

7. S.D. Hudson, "The Nature of Respect," *Social Theory and Practice* 6 (1980), pp. 69–90.

8. Warren, *Moral Status*, pp. 148–77.

9. L.J. Nelson and R.E. Cranford, "Michael Martin and Robert Wendland: Beyond the Vegetative State," *Journal of Contemporary Health Law and Policy* 15 (1999), pp. 427–53.

10. G. Annas, A. Caplan, and S. Elias, "The Politics of Human-Embryo Research—Avoiding Ethical Gridlock," *NEJM* 334 (1996), pp. 1329–32.

11. N. Tonti-Filippini, "The Catholic Church and Reproductive Technology," in *Bioethics: An Anthology*, ed. H. Kuhse and P. Singer (Malden, Mass.: Blackwell Publishers, 1999), pp. 93–95.

12. T.A. Shannon and A.B. Wolter, "Reflections on the Moral Status of the Pre-Embryo," *Theological Studies* 51 (1990), pp. 603–26.

13. N. Wade, "In the Ethics Storm on Human Embryo Research," *New York Times*, 28 September 1999.

14. A. Gutman and D. Thompson, *Democracy and Disagreement* (Cambridge, Mass.: Harvard University Press, 1996), pp. 52–94.

15. T.L. Beauchamp, "The Failure of Theories of Personhood," *Kennedy Institute of Ethics Journal* 9, no. 4 (1999), pp. 309–24.

16. Human Embryo Research Panel, *Final Report*, p. 47; CA. Tauer, "Embryo Research and Public Policy: A Philosopher's Appraisal," *The Journal of Medicine and Philosophy* 22 (1997), pp. 423–39.

17. A. Hultkrantz, *Belief and Worship in Native North America* (Syracuse: Syra-

cuse University Press, 1981), p. 120. See also C. Martin, *Keepers of the Game* (Berkeley, Calif.: University of California Press, 1978), pp. 113–49; D. Rockwell, *Giving Voice to Bear: North American Indian Rituals, Myths, and Images of the Bear* (Niwot, Co.: Robert Rinehart Publishers, 1991).

18. Martin, *Keepers*, p. 34.

19. Hultkrantz, *Belief and Worship*, p. 121; Martin, *Keepers*, pp. 18, 35–36; Rockwell, *Giving Voice*, p. 26.

20. Rockwell, *Giving Voice*, p. 33.

21. Martin, *Keepers*, p. 36.

22. Rockwell, *Giving Voice*, p. 38; Martin, *Keepers*, p. 36.

23. Martin, *Keepers*, p. 35; Hultkrantz, *Belief and Worship*, p. 122.

24. H. Hardacre, *Marketing the Menacing Fetus in Japan* (Berkeley: University of California Press, 1997), p. 2.

25. N. Wolf, "Our Bodies, Our Souls," in *The Abortion Controversy*, 2nd ed., ed. L. Pojman and F. Beckwith, (Belmont, Calif.: Wadsworth Publishing Company, 1998), p. 408.

26. T.C. Grey, *The Legal Enforcement of Morality* (New York: Alfred Knopf, 1983), p. 105.

27. D.G. Jones, *Speaking for the Dead* (Hants, England: Ashgate Pub., 2000), pp. 48, 49.

28. W.F. May, "Religion and the Donation of Body Parts," *Hastings Center Report* 15, no. 1 (1985), p. 39.

29. Jones, *Speaking*, p. 63.

30. A.Z. v. B.Z., 725 N.E.2d 1051 (Mass. 2000).

31. R.J. Levine, *Ethics and Regulation of Clinical Research*, 2nd ed. (Baltimore, Md.: Urban & Schwarzenberg, 1986), p. 3.

32. Human Embryo Research Panel, *Final Report*, p. ix.

33. R. McCormick, "Who or What Is the Preembryo?" *Kennedy Institute of Ethics Journal* 1 (1991), pp. 1–15; N.M. Ford, *When Did I Begin?* (Cambridge: Cambridge University Press, 1989).

3

Early Human Embryos Are Not Human Beings

Helga Kuhse and Peter Singer

Helga Kuhse is an associate professor in bioethics at Monash University in Clayton, Australia. Peter Singer is the DeCamp Professor of the Princeton University Center for Human Values. Kuhse and Singer are the editors of the book Embryo Experimentation, *from which this excerpt is taken.*

The major objections to early embryo human experimentation are problematic. One objection is that a newly fertilized egg is genetically unique as a human being. However, an early embryo may divide at a certain stage, become different cell groups, and become identical twins. The other objection rests on the claim that every human has a right to live. In actuality, the early embryo does not have the mental capacities of a human being, which supposedly set human beings apart from other organisms with lesser moral status. To protect human embryos from suffering, embryonic experimentation should not be conducted after embryos are twenty-eight days old, at which time they become sentient.

It is often assumed that the answer to the question: 'When does a particular human life begin?' will also provide the answer to the question of how that life ought, morally, to be treated. We shall, however, set the moral question aside for the moment and instead focus on some prior issues that must be faced by anyone who wants to claim that fertilization marks the time when a particular human life or 'I' began to exist.[1]

What this claim amounts to is that the newly fertilized egg, the early embryo and I are, in some sense of the term, the same individual. Now, in one very obvious sense, the zygote that gave rise to me and I, the adult, are not the same individual—the former is a unicellular being totally devoid of consciousness, whereas I am a conscious being consisting of many millions of cells. So the claim that the zygote and I are the same individual must rely on a different sense of 'individual'. And so it does.

It is usually thought that the zygote and I are the same individual in

Excerpted from *Embryo Experimentation*, by Helga Kuhse and Peter Singer (New York: Cambridge University Press, 1990). Copyright © 1990 by Cambridge University Press. Reprinted by permission of the authors.

one or both of the following two senses: first, that there is a genetic continuity between the zygote and me (we share the same genetic code); and, second, that there is what, for want of a better term, one might call 'numerical continuity' between us (we are the same single thing). In other words, the zygote does not just have the potential to produce an as-yet-unidentifiable individual, rather the zygote is, from the first moment of its existence, already a particular individual—Tom, or Dick, or Harry. But, as we shall see, this view, which we shall call the 'identity thesis', faces some very serious problems. For, contrary to what is often believed, recent scientific findings do not support the view that fertilization marks the event when a particular, identifiable individual begins to exist.

It is true that the life of the fertilized ovum is a genetically new life in the sense that it is neither genetically nor numerically continuous with the life of the egg or the sperm before fertilization. Before fertilization, there were two genetically distinct entities, the egg and the sperm; now there is only one entity, the fertilized egg or zygote, with a new and unique genetic code. It is also true that the zygote will—other things being equal—develop into an embryo, fetus and baby with the same genetic code.

Problems with the identity thesis

But, as we shall see, things are not always equal and some serious problems are raised for supporters of the identity thesis.

Here are two scenarios of what might happen during early human development.

In the first scenario, a man and a woman have intercourse, fertilization takes place, and a genetically new zygote, let's call it Tom, is formed. Tom has a specific genetic identity—a genetic blueprint—that will be repeated in every cell once the first cell begins to split, first into two, then into four cells, and so on. On day 8, however, the group of cells which is Tom divides into two separate identical cell groups. These two separate cell groups continue to develop and, some nine months later, identical twins are born. Now, which one, if either of them, is Tom? There are no obvious grounds for thinking of one of the twins as Tom and the other as Not-Tom; the twinning process is quite symmetrical and both twins have the same genetic blueprint as the original Tom. But to suggest that both of them are Tom does, of course, conflict with numerical continuity: there was one zygote and now there are two babies.

People have thought in various ways about this: for example, that when the original cell split, Tom ceased to exist and that two new individuals, Dick and Harry, came into existence. But if that were conceded then it would, of course, no longer be true that the existence of the babies Dick and Harry began at fertilization: their existence did not begin until eight days *after* fertilization. Moreover (and we shall come back to this in a moment) if Tom died on day 8, how is it that he left no earthly remains?

Now consider the second scenario. A man and a woman have intercourse and fertilization takes place. But this time, two eggs are fertilized and two zygotes come into existence—Mary and Jane. The zygotes begin to divide, first into two, then into four cells, and so on. But, then, on day 6, the two embryos combine, forming what is known as a chimera, and continue to develop as a single organism, which will eventually become a baby. Now, who is the baby—Mary or Jane, both Mary and Jane, or somebody else—Nancy?

In one plausible sense of the term, there is genetic continuity between Mary, Jane and the baby. Because the baby is a chimera, she carries the unique genetic code of both Mary and Jane. Some of the millions of cells that make up her body contain the genetic code of Mary, others the genetic code of Jane. So in that sense the baby would seem to be both Mary and Jane. But in terms of numerical continuity, this poses a problem. There is now only one individual where there were formerly two. Does this mean that Mary or Jane, or both of them, have ceased to exist? But to suggest that one of them has ceased to exist poses the problem of explaining why one and not the other should have ceased to exist. Moreover, to say that anyone has ceased to exist will put one in the difficult position (already encountered in the previous example of Tom) of having to explain how it can be that a human individual has ceased to exist when nothing has been lost or has perished—in other words, when there has been a death but there is no corpse.

We could sketch other scenarios to show further complexities, but enough has been said to demonstrate that even before the advent of new reproductive technologies serious problems were raised for the 'identity thesis'. As we shall see, these problems have been compounded by new scientific findings.

It is now believed that early embryonic cells are totipotent; that is, that, contrary to the 'identity thesis', an early human embryo is not one particular individual, but rather has the potential to become one or more different individuals. Up to the 8-cell stage, each single embryonic cell is a distinct entity in the sense that there is no fusion between the individual cells; rather, the embryo is a loose collection of distinct cells, held together by the zona pellucida, the outer membrane of the egg. Animal studies on four-cell embryos indicate that each one of these cells has the potential to produce at least one fetus or baby.

Recent scientific findings do not support the view that fertilization marks the event when a particular, identifiable individual begins to exist.

Take a human embryo consisting of four cells. On the assumption that this embryo is a particular human individual, we shall call it Adam. Because each of Adam's four cells is totipotent, any three cells could be removed from the zona pellucida and the remaining cell would still have the potential to develop into a perfect fetus or baby. Now, it might be thought that this baby is Adam, the same baby that would have resulted had all four cells continued to develop jointly. But this poses a problem because we could have left any one of the other three cells in the zona pellucida, each with the potential to develop into a baby. The same baby—Adam? Things are not made any easier by the recognition that the three 'surplus' cells, each placed into an empty zona pellucida, would also have the potential to develop into babies. We now have four distinct human individuals with the potential to develop into four babies. Because it does not make good sense to identify any one particular individual as Adam, let's call them Bill, Charles, David and Eddy.

This example shows that there are not only problems regarding individual identity, but also closely related problems regarding the early embryo's potential to produce one or more human individuals. In the above example, the zygote had the potential to produce either one individual, Adam, or four individuals—Bill, Charles, David and Eddy. But this is not where its potential ends. Had we waited until the embryo had cleaved one more time in its petri dish, there would have been not four, but eight, totipotent cells—that is, eight distinct individual entities oriented towards further development and hence eight potential babies: Fred, Graeme, Harry, Ivan and so on. Moreover, since these individual cells also have the potential to recombine to form, say, just one or two distinct individuals, fertilization cannot be regarded as the beginning of a particular human life.

An early human embryo is not one particular individual, but rather has the potential to become one or more different individuals.

Those who want to object to embryo experimentation because it destroys a particular or identifiable human life would be on much safer ground were they to argue that a particular human life begins not at fertilization but at around day 14 after fertilization. By that time, totipotency has been lost, and the development of the primitive streak precludes the embryo from becoming two or more different individuals through twinning. Once the primitive streak has formed, it would thus be much easier to argue that it is Adam, Bill or Charles that is developing, or all three of them, but as distinct individuals.

The standard argument

Next we want to raise the moral question that we set aside at the beginning of this chapter. Let us assume that we have settled the issue of when a particular individual's life begins—and for the moment it doesn't matter whether this happens at around day 14 or at fertilization. All that we need to assume for our present purposes is that there is such a marker event, that we have identified it and that the entity we are talking about has crossed this particular developmental hurdle.

Now what is it about the new human entity that could raise moral questions about destructive embryo experimentation? Many people believe that it is wrong to use human embryos in research because these embryos are human beings, and all human beings have a right to life. The syllogism goes like this:

Every human being has a right to life.
A human embryo is a human being.
Therefore the human embryo has a right to life.

In case anyone is worrying about issues like capital punishment, or killing in self-defence, we should perhaps add that the term 'innocent' is here and henceforth assumed whenever we are talking of human beings and their rights.

The standard argument has a standard response: to accept the first premise—that all human beings have a right to life—but to deny the second premise, that the human embryo is a human being. This standard response, however, runs into difficulties, because the embryo is clearly a being, of some sort, and it can't possibly be of any other species than *Homo sapiens*. Thus it seems to follow that it must be a human being.

Questioning the first premise

So the standard argument for attributing a right to life to the embryo can withstand the standard response. It is not easy to challenge directly the claim that the embryo is a human being. What the standard argument cannot withstand, however, is a more critical examination of its first premise: that every human being has a right to life. At first glance, this seems the stronger premise. Do we really want to deny that every (innocent) human being has a right to life? Are we about to condone murder? No wonder it is on the second premise that most of the fire has been directed. But the surprising vulnerability of the first premise becomes apparent as soon as we cease to take 'Every human being has a right to life' as an unquestionable moral axiom, and instead inquire into the moral basis for our particular objection to killing human beings.

By 'our particular objection to killing human beings', we mean the objection we have to killing human beings, over and above any objection we have to killing other living beings, such as pigs and cows and dogs and cats, and even trees and lettuces. Why do we think killing human beings is so much more serious than killing these other beings?

The obvious answer is that human beings are different from other animals, and the greater seriousness of killing them is a result of these differences. But which of the many differences between humans and other animals justify such a distinction? Again, the obvious response is that the morally relevant differences are those based on our superior mental powers—our self-awareness, our rationality, our moral sense, our autonomy, or some combination of these. They are the kinds of thing, we are inclined to say, which make us 'uniquely human'. To be more precise, they are the kinds of thing which make us persons.

That the particular objection to killing human beings rests on such qualities is very plausible. To take the most extreme of the differences between living things, consider a person who is enjoying life, is part of a network of relationships with other people, is looking forward to what tomorrow may bring, and is freely choosing the course her or his life will take for the years to come. Now think about a lettuce, which, we can safely assume, knows and feels nothing at all. One would have to be quite mad, or morally blind, or warped, not to see that killing the person is far more serious than killing the lettuce.

We shall postpone asking which mental qualities make it more morally serious to kill a person than to kill a lettuce. For our immediate purposes, we will merely note that the plausibility of the assertion that human beings have a right to life depends on the fact that human beings generally possess mental qualities that other living beings do not possess.

So should we accept the premise that every human being has a right to life? We may do so, but only if we bear in mind that by 'human being' here we refer to those beings who have the mental qualities which generally distinguish members of our species from members of other species.

If this is the sense in which we can accept the first premise, however, what of the second premise? It is immediately clear that in the sense of the term 'human being' which is required to make the first premise acceptable, the second premise is false. The embryo, especially the early embryo, is obviously not a being with the mental qualities that generally distinguish members of our species from members of other species. The early embryo has no brain, no nervous system. It is reasonable to assume that, so far as its mental life goes, it has no more awareness than a lettuce.

It is still true that the human embryo is a member of the species *Homo sapiens*. That is why it is difficult to deny that the human embryo is a human being. But we can now see that this is not the sense of 'human being' needed to make the standard argument work. A valid argument cannot equivocate on the meanings of its central terms. If the first premise is true when 'human' means 'a being with certain mental qualities' and the second premise is true when 'human' means 'member of the species *Homo sapiens*', the argument is based on a slide between the two meanings, and is invalid.

The sense in which the embryo is a human being is not the sense in which we should accept that every human being has a right to life.

Can the argument be rescued? It obviously can't be rescued by claiming that the embryo is a being with the requisite mental qualities. That might be arguable only for some later stage of the development of the fetus. If the second premise cannot be reconciled with the first, then, can the first perhaps be defended in a form which makes it compatible with the second? Can it be argued that human beings have a right to life, not because of any moral qualities they may possess, but because they—unlike pigs, cows, dogs or lettuces—are members of the species *Homo sapiens*?

This is a desperate move. Those who make it find themselves having to defend the claim that species membership is in itself morally relevant to the wrongness of killing a being. But why should that be so? If we are considering whether it is wrong to destroy something, surely we must look at its actual characteristics, not just the species to which it belongs. If visitors from other planets turn out to be sensitive, thinking, planning beings, who form deep and lasting relationships just like we do, would it be acceptable to kill them simply because they are not members of our species? What if we substituted 'race' for 'species' in the question? If we reject the claim that membership of a particular race is in itself morally relevant to the wrongness of killing a being, it is not easy to see how we could accept the same claim when based on species membership. The fact that other races, like our own, can feel, think and plan for the future is not relevant to this question, for we are considering membership in a particular group—whether race or species—as the sole basis for determining the wrongness of killing members of one group or another. It seems clear that neither race nor species can, in itself, provide any justifiable basis for such a distinction.

So the standard argument fails. It does so not because the embryo is not a human being, but because the sense in which the embryo is a human being is not the sense in which we should accept that every human being has a right to life.

The Golden Rule

We have now seen the inadequacies of arguing that the human zygote or early embryo is a distinct human individual, and that destructive embryo experimentation is wrong because the zygote or embryo is a member of the human species. But there are other reasons why one might consider embryo experimentation wrong. Since the early embryo, devoid of a nervous system or a brain, can neither experience pain or pleasure, nor any of the things occurring in the world, the most important thing about it is that it is a potential baby or person, a person just like us. In other words, when we destroy an early human embryo in research, a potential baby or person will now not exist.

Why is this fact morally significant? One plausible answer is provided by R.M. Hare when he appeals, in a well-known article on abortion, to a type of formal argument, captured in the ancient Christian and pre-Christian Golden Rule, that has been the basis of almost all theories of moral reasoning: that we should do to others as we wish them to do to us.[2] In other words, given that we are glad that nobody destroyed us when we were embryos, we should, other things being equal, not destroy an embryo that would have a life like us.

We believe the minimal characteristic needed to give the embryo a claim to consideration is sentience, or the capacity to feel pleasure or pain.

It might seem that the Golden Rule applied to embryo experimentation would impose on us an extremely conservative position, for it would seem to rule out the destruction of all but the most seriously abnormal zygote or embryo. But before we too readily embrace that conclusion, we should also note something already pointed out by Hare in the abortion context: when you are glad that you exist, you do not confine this gladness to gladness that you were not aborted when an embryo or fetus. Rather, you are also glad that you were brought into existence in the first place—that your parents had intercourse without contraception when they did.[3]

Let us apply this sort of thinking to our present context—that of the in vitro fertilization (IVF) embryo—and assume that, at some time between the beginning of the process of fertilization and the formation of the primitive streak, the existence of an identifiable individual began. Let us also assume that you developed from that individual. Now, it will immediately become apparent that regardless of what event marked the beginning of your life as an identifiable entity, none of the other events that preceded it were any less important for your present existence. Just as you would not have existed had a scientist performed a destructive experiment on the embryo from which you developed when it was 14 days old, so you would not have existed had she or he performed it on the zygote when it was one day old. Similarly, you would not have existed had your mother's egg with your father's sperm already inside it been destroyed just before syngamy had occurred, or just after that event. Nor, we should hasten to add, would you have existed had the scientist, instead of using one particular egg, used another egg or had a different sperm fertilized the egg, and so on.

The upshot is that the marker event for the beginning of a human individual, on whose identification so much time and energy is being expended, is of no importance so far as the existence of a particular person is concerned. If it is the existence of a particular person that is relevant—a Tom, a Dick, or a Harry—who would treasure his life in much the same way as we do, then it does not matter whether his existence was thwarted before or after fertilization, or the formation of the primitive streak, had occurred.

The [non-sentient human] embryo ranks, morally, with . . . non-human animals.

We should also note that there are numerous ways in which the existence of particular individuals can be thwarted. A totipotent IVF embryo, for example, is not, as we saw, one particular individual, but rather an entity with the potential to become one or more different individuals, because each cell is a distinct entity with the potential for further development. What are we doing, then, when we refrain from separating the cells, leaving all four or eight of them together? And what are we doing when we extract and destroy a single cell for gene-typing of the embryo? We believe we should, in consistency, say that we are depriving a number of human individuals of their chance of existence.

This is one important point. The other important point is this: our reproductive choices almost invariably constitute an explicit or implicit choice between different individuals. We said a moment ago that had the scientist who assisted your imaginary IVF conception used a different sperm or a different egg, you would not have existed, and the same thing applies, of course, to other scenarios in natural reproduction as well. But—and this is the morally important point—seeing that your parents wanted to raise a child of their own, it is likely that another child would have been born. While this person would not have been you, it would have been a person just like you in the morally relevant sense that she or he would now, presumably, be just as glad to exist as you are glad to exist.

But if our reproductive choices typically constitute a choice between different individuals, then the destruction of early human embryos—particularly if it makes possible improved IVF techniques and, therefore, the existence of IVF children who would not otherwise have existed—is no harder to justify than many of our other reproductive choices: for example, when and with whom, to have intercourse, without contraception, to have the two or three children we are going to have.

Flawed objections

We have now seen that some of the most common objections to destructive experimentation on early human embryos are seriously flawed. But when, in its development from zygote to baby, does the embryo acquire any rights or interests? We believe the minimal characteristic needed to give the embryo a claim to consideration is sentience, or the capacity to feel pleasure or pain. Until that point is reached, the embryo does not have any interests and, like other non-sentient organisms (a human egg, for example), cannot be harmed—in a morally relevant sense—by anything we do. We can, of course, damage the embryo in such a way as to cause harm to the sentient being it will become, if it lives, but if it never becomes a sentient being, the embryo has not been harmed, because its total lack of awareness means that it never has had any interests at all.

The fact that the early embryo has no interests is also relevant to a distinction embodied in the *Infertility (Medical Procedures) Act 1984* between 'spare' embryos left over from infertility treatments (which may be used in experimentation), and the creation of embryos especially for research (which is prohibited).[4] The report of the Waller Committee [formally known as the In Vitro Fertilisation Committee, which is based in Australia], on which the legislation is based, speaks of such a creation as using a human being as a means rather than as an end.[5] This is a principle of Kantian ethics that makes some sense when applied to rational, autonomous beings—or perhaps even, though more controversially, when applied to sentient beings who, though not rational or autonomous, may have ends of their own. There is no basis at all, however, for applying it to a totally non-sentient embryo, which can have no ends of its own.

Finally, we point to a curious consequence of restrictive legislation on embryo research. In sharp contrast to the human embryo at this early stage of its existence, non-human animals such as primates, dogs, rabbits, guinea pigs, rats and mice clearly can feel pain, and thus often are harmed by what is done to them in the course of scientific research. We have already suggested that the species of a being is not, in itself, relevant to its ethical status. Why, then, is it considered acceptable to poison conscious rabbits in order to test the safety of drugs and household chemicals, but not considered acceptable to carry out tests on totally non-sentient human embryos? It is only when an embryo reaches the stage at which it may be capable of feeling pain that we need to control the experimentation which can be done with it. At this point the embryo ranks, morally, with those non-human animals we have mentioned. These animals have often been unjustifiably made to suffer in scientific research. We should have stringent controls over research to ensure that this cannot happen to embryos, just as we should have stringent controls to ensure that it cannot happen to animals.

At what point, then, does the embryo develop a capacity to feel pain? Though we are not experts in this field, from our reading of the literature, we would say that it cannot possibly be earlier than six weeks, and it may well be as late as 18 or 20 weeks.[6] While we think we should err on the side of caution, it seems to us that the 14-day limit suggested by both the Waller and Warnock committees is too conservative.[7] [The Warnock Committee is formally known as the Inquiry into Embryology, which is based in Australia.] There is no doubt that the embryo is not sentient for some time after this date. Even if we were to be very, very cautious in erring on the safe side, a 28-day limit would provide sufficient protection against the possibility of an embryo suffering during experimentation.

Notes

1. For a more detailed discussion of this issue, see Norman Ford, *When Did I Begin?* (Cambridge University Press, Cambridge, 1988).

2. Hare, R.M., "Abortion and the Golden Rule," *Philosophy and Public Affairs* 4: 3 (1975), pp. 201–22.

3. Ibid, p. 212.

4. *Infertility (Medical Procedures) Act 1984* (Vic.).

5. Committee to Consider the Social, Ethical and Legal Issues Arising from In Vitro Fertilization, *Report on the Disposition of Embryos Produced by In Vitro Fertilization* (Prof. Louis Waller, chairman), (Victorian Government Printer, Melbourne, 1984), para. 3.27.

6. For an expert opinion on when a fetus may begin to be capable of feeling pain, see the report of the British Government's Advisory Group on Fetal Research, *The Use of Foetuses and Foetal Material for Research* (Sir John Peel, chairman), (HMSO, London, 1972). A clear summary of some relevant scientific evidence, with further references, can be found in M. Tooley, *Abortion and Infanticide* (Clarendon Press, Oxford, 1983), pp. 347–407.

7. Waller, op. cit., para. 3.29; and *Report of the Committee of Inquiry into Human Fertilization and Embryology* (Mary Warnock, chair), (HMSO, London, 1984), pars. 11.19–11.22.

4

Embryonic Stem Cell Research Should Be Federally Funded

Lawrence S.B. Goldstein

Lawrence S.B. Goldstein is a professor in the Department of Cellular and Molecular Medicine at the University of California, San Diego, School of Medicine and a Howard Hughes Medical Institute investigator.

Decades of scientific research show the potential benefits of embryonic stem (ES) cell research. ES cells—which are derived from early-stage human embryos—may have the ability to generate many types of replacement cells and tissues to help treat diseases which are the result of cell or tissue malfunction. Although stem cells derived from adult tissue present exciting possibilities, it is too early to conclude that the potential use of adult stem cells eliminates the need for further ES cell research. Therefore, ES research needs to be supported by federal funds to ensure that all the possibilities of this new medical technology are explored.

The [George W.] Bush administration is deeply divided over whether to permit the use of taxpayer funds to pay for research using embryonic stem cells. At issue is whether a particular area of biomedical research that can potentially save many lives and could ease suffering in years to come should be limited because of the ethical concerns and religious beliefs of some of our citizens. [Bush has permitted stem cell research to receive limited federal support.]

Each one of us, including the president, must make a decision about this issue that balances information from scientific data, medical need, diverse ethical values and the public interest. To make an informed decision, however, it is essential that we have clear and accurate information.

There are four major issues about which there has been substantial confusion about the facts, but which are critical to making a decision about public funding of stem cell research.

First is the question of whether the scientific data allow a decision to

Excerpted from "Stem Cell Research: For Balancing Benefits, Ethical Values," by Lawrence S.B. Goldstein, *The San Diego Union-Tribune*, July 6, 2001. Copyright © 2001 by *The San Diego Union-Tribune*. Reprinted by permission of the author.

be made on the potential and value of research on so-called adult stem cells relative to embryonic stem cells. Embryonic stem cells are derived from early stage embryos when they are a hollow ball of 50-100 cells. These cells appear to have the capacity to become any adult tissue or cell type, hence the interest in their potential to treat diseases such as Alzheimer's, diabetes and many others.

Adults are also known to have stem cells in some tissues. Until recently, cells from adults were thought to have only limited potential to make different cell types, and hence thought to have only limited utility to treat disease, with bone marrow transplant being the only notable success. Some recent research has suggested that adult cells might have a greater capacity than originally thought, and this has led a few scientists to suggest that adult stem cells might have equivalent therapeutic potential to embryonic stem cells.

At issue is whether a particular area of biomedical research that can potentially save many lives . . . should be limited because of the ethical concerns and religious beliefs of some of our citizens.

While this is an exciting possibility, most of the top scientists working on adult stem cells, including most of those whose studies are cited by opponents of embryonic stem cell research, have stated that while their research is very promising, it would be a mistake to conclude research on embryonic cells is unnecessary. In addition, we have decades of data and thousands of published experiments that establish the potential of embryonic stem cells.

The experiments that are interpreted to mean that adult stem cells have equivalent properties to embryonic cells have in most cases been done only recently, are often single experiments that have not been demonstrated to have a high degree of reliability and reproducibility, and are characterized in some cases by indirect or limited data that are used to support broad conclusions.

It would be a mistake to base important policy decisions affecting the health and lives of many of our citizens upon such an incomplete and immature body of data.

Second is the question of whether it is possible to be pro-life and to still favor public funding of embryonic stem cell research. The facts are clear: embryonic stem cell research is supported by many prominent citizens and legislators such as former Senator Connie Mack, current Senators Strom Thurmond, John McCain, Orrin Hatch and Gordon Smith and Rep. Randy "Duke" Cunningham of Escondido, California.

These men are all ethical, religious, anti-abortion Republicans who recognize that for a variety of sensible reasons, in vitro fertilization procedures sometimes generate more embryos than are needed for treatment of infertility. These embryos are sometimes legally and ethically discarded when there is no longer clinical need for them, usually after they have been stored frozen for several years.

These legislators, and many other citizens who oppose abortions, realize that it makes no sense to discard frozen human embryos without regard to the possible benefit of obtaining stem cells for potentially life-saving research. To quote Hatch from his recent letter to President Bush: "After carefully analyzing the factors involved, I conclude that, at this time, research on human pluripotent embryonic stem cells is legal, scientifically compelling, and ethically sound."

Third is the question of whether morality, ethics and decency demand that the early human embryo be afforded the same legal and ethical protections that we give to adult humans. While some religious traditions such as Greek orthodox, some branches of fundamentalist Christianity, and the official Roman Catholic position assert that the human zygote or early embryo before implantation is entitled to full protection as an adult human, other religious traditions such as Judaism, Islam, Presbyterianism and some other Christian denominations do not share this view.

In fact, the suggestion that an early human embryo composed of 50–100 cells, and which has no heart, no blood, no brain and no human features other than a human genome, is entitled to the same legal and ethical protections that we give to adult humans is unprecedented and not embodied in American law. To quote Hatch from his letter to Health and Human Services Secretary Tommy Thompson, "In evaluating this issue, it is significant to point out that no member of the United States Supreme Court has ever taken the position that fetuses, let alone embryos, are constitutionally protected persons. As much as I oppose partial birth abortion, I simply cannot equate this offensive abortion practice with the act of disposing of a frozen embryo in the case where the embryo will never complete the journey toward birth. Nor, for example, can I imagine Congress or the courts somehow attempting to order every 'spare' embryo through a full-term pregnancy."

The need for public funding

Finally, there is the question of whether public funding is needed in view of the interest in this area from private industry. In fact, private industry will put the bulk of its resources where there is the greatest profit potential. Still, there are many diseases where embryonic stem cell therapies may be important, but where there is not sufficient profit potential or competitive advantage to warrant the needed risk, investment and effort.

Private industry is also unlikely to do the large amount of basic research on the properties of embryonic cells that will be needed to understand why these cells are special and how we might induce other non-embryonic cells such as adult stem cells to acquire these properties. Granted, private industry will continue to work in this area without public funding. But, the work will go more slowly, and it will likely occur with only limited, if any, public input into the ethics and conduct of the work.

People of good conscience can disagree on these issues and may weigh these arguments differently. It is important however, to know the facts before deciding, especially when they are so clear.

5

Cloning Human Embryos for Therapeutic Purposes Should Be Allowed

Michael D. West

Michael D. West is president and chief executive officer of Advanced Cell Technology, a biotechnology company based in Worcester, Massachusetts.

Finding a humane and practical means of meeting America's growing health care needs may depend on the advancement of embryonic stem (ES) cell technology. Stem cells derived from early-staged human embryos have the potential to generate a wide range of human tissues for transplantation. As encouraging as stem cell technology may be, the high probability that an individual's body will reject transplanted tissues remains a challenge. However, if an individual has embryos cloned from his or her own cells, tissues and organs could be created specifically for that individual through ES technology. Therefore, research into cloning early-staged human embryos for therapeutic purposes should continue.

I am pleased to testify in regard to the new opportunities and challenges associated with human embryonic stem (ES) cell and nuclear transfer (NT) technologies. By way of introduction, I believe it is important to bring to mind the context of these new opportunities. We are approaching a period in our national history of unparalleled growth of the elderly sector of the population. The aging of the baby boom population along with a general increase in the number of aged people is expected to increase the number of the elderly sevenfold between 1980 and 2030 A.D. And since the aged use a disproportionately high percentage of health care, this "graying of America" is likely to greatly strain our national resources. It has been estimated that transplantation procedures currently account for nearly half of our health care expenditures, approaching $400 billion annually. This is likely to grow even larger with the aging of our population and result in a marked increase in the demand for transplantation. The increased incidence of age-related degenerative disease will

Excerpted from Michael D. West's testimony to the Science, Technology, and Space Subcommittee on Labor, Health and Human Services, and Education. December 2, 1998.

likely lead to conflicts of economics, ethics, and aesthetics as we struggle to find a humane and practical means of treating the ailing. Concrete examples of tissues needed will likely include: heart tissue for heart failure, arrhythmias, and ischemic damage; cartilage for arthritis; neurons for Parkinson's disease; kidney cells for kidney failure; liver cells for cirrhosis and hepatitis; skin for burns and ulcers; and bone marrow transplantations for cancer to name only a few. While current procedures are partially successful in alleviating human suffering, these procedures are limited by two major difficulties: 1) the availability of the needed cell or tissue type, and 2) the histocompatibility of the transplanted tissues [which determines whether the body will ultimately reject the transplanted tissue]. As a result, thousands of patients die every year for the lack of transplantable cells and tissues, and projections from the Bureau of the Census suggest this shortage will worsen with the aging of our population.

Human ES cells

Human ES cell technologies may greatly improve the availability of diverse cell types. Human ES cells are unique in that they stand near the base of the developmental tree. These cells are frequently designated "totipotent" stem cells, meaning that they are potentially capable of forming any cell or tissue type needed in medicine. These differ from previously-isolated stem cells that are "pluripotent," that is, capable of forming several, but only a limited number, of cell types. An example of pluripotent stem cells are the bone marrow stem cells now widely used in the treatment of cancer and other life-threatening diseases.

With appropriate funding of research, we may soon learn to direct these cells to become vehicles of lifesaving potential. We may, for instance, become able to produce neurons for the treatment of Parkinson's disease and spinal cord injury, heart muscle cells for heart failure, cartilage for arthritis and many others as well. This research has great potential to help solve the first problem of tissue availability, but the technologies to direct these cells to become various cell types in adequate quantities remains to be elucidated. Because literally hundreds of cell types are needed, thousands of academic research projects need to be funded, far exceeding the resources of the biotechnology industry.

As promising as ES cell technology may be, it does not solve the second problem of histocompatibility. Human ES cells obtained from embryos derived during in vitro fertilization procedures, or from fetal sources, are essentially cells from another individual (allogeneic). Several approaches can be envisioned to solve the problem of histocompatibility. One approach would be to make vast numbers of human ES cell lines that could be stored in a frozen state. This "library" of cells would then offer varied surface antigens, such that the patient's physician could search through the library for cells that are as close as possible to the patient. But these would likely still require simultaneous immunosuppression that is not always effective. In addition, immunosuppressive therapy carries with it increased cost, and the risk of complications including malignancy and even death.

Another theoretical solution would be to genetically modify the cultured ES cells to make them "universal donor" cells. That is, the cells would have genes added or genes removed that would "mask" the foreign nature of the cells, allowing the patient's immune system to see the cells as "self." While such technologies may be developed in the future, it is also possible that these technologies may carry with them unacceptably high risks of rejection or other complications that would limit their practical utility in clinical practice.

Given the seriousness of the current shortage of transplantable cells and tissues, the Food and Drug Administration (FDA) has demonstrated a willingness to consider a broad array of options including the sourcing of cells and indeed whole organs from animals (xenografts) although these sources also pose unique problems of histocompatibility. These animal cells do have the advantage that they have the potential to be genetically engineered to approach the status of "universal donor" cells, through genetic engineering. However as described above, no simple procedure to confer such universal donor status is known. Most such procedures are still experimental and would likely continue to require the use of drugs to hold off rejection, drugs that add to health care costs, and carry the risk of life-threatening complications.

Therapeutic cloning

A promising solution to this remaining problem of histocompatibility would be to create human ES cells genetically identical to the patient. While no ES cells are known to exist in a developed human being and are therefore not available for treatment, such cells could possibly be obtained through the procedure of somatic cell nuclear transfer (NT). In this still largely theoretical procedure, body cells from a patient would be fused with an egg cell that has had its nucleus (including the nuclear DNA) removed. This would theoretically allow the production of a blastocyst-staged embryo genetically identical to the patient that could, in turn, lead to the production of ES cells identical to the patient. In addition, published data suggests that the procedure of NT can "rejuvenate" an aged cell, restoring the proliferative capacity inherent in cells at the beginning of life. Therefore, NT as applied to the production of therapeutic stem cells could have valuable and important applications in the treatment of age-related degenerative diseases.

Human ES cell technologies may greatly improve the availability of diverse cell types. . . . They are potentially capable of forming any cell or tissue type needed in medicine.

The use of somatic cell nuclear transfer for the purposes of dedifferentiating a patient's cells for purposes of obtaining undifferentiated stem cells has been designated "Therapeutic Cloning" in the United Kingdom. This terminology is used to differentiate this clinical indication from the use of NT for the cloning of a child which in turn is designated "Reproductive Cloning" in the United Kingdom. In the United Kingdom, the use of NT for therapeutic cloning is being encouraged while legislation has been passed to prohibit reproductive cloning.

As promising as NT technologies may be in the arena of therapeutic cloning, a remaining difficulty would be on a source of human oocytes, both for research purposes, but also eventually for large-scale clinical implementation. We believe there may be certain advantages to the use of "surrogate" oocytes from animal sources. Animal oocytes could be supplied in large numbers on an economical basis, they could be "humanized" so as to provide fully human cells with human, rather than animal, mitochondria, and they could also potentially be engineered to be defective in producing a fetus even if used in an inappropriate effort to clone a human being by implantation in a uterus. Since these oocytes would be produced in cloned animals (presumably cows), they could, in principle, offer two advantages: 1) an economical and ethically acceptable source of oocytes for therapeutic cloning, and 2) it is possible that they could be engineered to be effective in dedifferentiating human cells and allowing differentiation into specific lineages, but defective in creating a human embryo if implanted into a uterus. This may prevent the abuse of the technology in the event of an inappropriate use of the technology in attempting to produce a pregnancy.

The NT technologies described above are not designed to be used for the cloning of a human being. [The biotechnology company] Advanced Cell Technology has no intent to clone a human being, and we are opposed to efforts to clone a human being. As of today, we see no clear utility in producing a child by NT, and even if such uses were identified, NT would likely carry with it an inappropriately high risk of embryonic and fetal wastage. However, we believe that the production of genetically-engineered surrogate animal oocytes may be an important resource for medical research, and may solve certain practical and ethical problems associated with sourcing human oocytes and the risks of abuse in human reproductive cloning.

It should be emphasized that the above-mentioned technologies are still in the very earliest stages of development. It is not possible as of today to determine whether the production of human ES cells through sexual or asexual means will meet all the necessary requirements for the development of human therapeutics. What is clear however, is that a careful, informed, and reasoned public discourse would help insure that these technologies could develop to the point where they could be used in the clinic to treat human disease.

Ethical considerations

The problem of sourcing human cells and tissues for transplantation raises numerous ethical dilemmas. Because developing embryonic and fetal cells and tissues are "young" and are still in the process of forming mature tissues, there has been considerable interest in obtaining these tissues for use in human medicine. However, the use of aborted embryo or fetal tissue raises numerous issues ranging from concerns over increasing the frequency of elected abortion, to simple issues of maintaining quality controls standards in this hypothetical industry. Similarly, obtaining cells and tissues from living donors or cadavers is also not without ethical issues. For instance, an important and largely unresolved issue is whether it is morally acceptable to keep "deceased" individuals on life support for long periods of time in order to harvest organs as they are needed.

The implementation of ES-based technologies could address some of the ethical problems described above. First, it is important to note that the production of large numbers of human ES cells would not in itself cause these same concerns in accessing human embryonic or fetal tissue, since the resulting cells have the potential to be grown for very long periods of time. Using only a limited number of human embryos not used during in vitro fertilization procedures, biotechnology could theoretically supply the needs of many millions of patients if the problem of histocompatibility could be resolved. Second, in the case of NT procedures, the patient may be at lower risk of complications in transplant rejection. Third, the only human cells used would be from the patient. Theoretically, the need to access tissue from other human beings could be reduced.

A promising solution to this remaining problem of histocompatibility [the body's possible rejection of transplanted tissues] would be to create human ES cells genetically identical to the patient.

On March 4, 1997 [former] President Bill Clinton asked for a "moratorium on the cloning of human beings until our Bioethics Advisory Commission and our entire nation have had a real chance to understand and debate the profound ethical implications of the latest advances." Prior to this 1997 request and the cloning of Dolly [the first mammal to be created through a somatic cell nuclear transfer], Advanced Cell Technology had initiated research into the use of human somatic cell NT for human cell therapy (therapeutic cloning) and had obtained preliminary results that suggested the technology would be useful in treating disease. Following the President's request, however, the Company tabled all research in this area awaiting clarification of recommended guidelines. After internal review in 1998, the Company decided that it did not have sufficient data to assemble a scientific publication, but believed that it was in the public interest to release the preliminary results to promote an informed and reasoned public discussion of the issues. In this regard, we are grateful for the President's request of November 14, 1998 asking the National Bioethics Advisory Commission to analyze the issues surrounding this new technology.

Mixing DNA across species

In regard to the President's letter of November 14, 1998, we would like to offer the following observations. First, we share the President's concerns regarding the mixing of DNA across species. By way of background, it is useful to recall the debate surrounding the specter of mingling of human and non-human DNA in gene splicing technologies in the 1970s. In addition to the general discomfort of combining the genes of organisms across the plant and animal kingdoms, there were more focused concerns raised concerning the deliberate mixing of the genomes of viruses such as adenovirus and tumor viruses such as SV40 or between SV40 and bacteria such as E. coli for fear that new and virulent man-made pathogens may unintentionally result in a major health risk. Shortly thereafter, there were again concerns voiced over the mixing of antibiotic resistance genes in bacteria not then possessing such resistance. The resolution of those concerns may guide us in the consideration of these new technologies. The use of attenuated strains of host organism and other precautions have served us well and allowed recombinant technology to advance and, in doing so, to improve the human condition.

Concerns over the mixing of the genomes of differing species is even of greater concern given newer technologies that allow the transfer of entire chromosomes across species. Given justifiable concerns that these technologies not be abused in medical research, we join in asking for ethical debate of the issue of the mixing of genomic DNA across species.

The mixing of DNA across species does not, however, bear on the issue of NT. The research performed in 1996 resulted in human cells with less than one millionth of the DNA being from a nonhuman (bovine) source, and that DNA was for the mitochondria, an energy source for the cell, not encoding species-specific traits such as eye color, intelligence, or other distinctive features. In addition, it was, and is, the intent of Advanced Cell Technology to produce fully-human stem cells through the genetic modification of the bovine egg cell to introduce human mitochondrial DNA.

Seeking guidelines

The relevant issue is that the biotechnology industry is seeking guidelines for the application of ES and NT technologies in medicine. We believe that these new technologies, if properly applied, could lead to significant medical advances with lifesaving potential. Poorly constructed legislation, designed to prohibit the cloning of a human being, could inadvertently interfere with urgent and ethical applications of the technologies in medicine.

Prohibitions against humanized surrogate NT may also have serious collateral consequences in addition to harming these new therapeutic avenues. During various in vitro protocols, it is not unlikely that human oocytes or embryos may be cultured in the presence of bovine proteins, such as bovine fetal calf serum. It would be unwise to set a precedent that the contact of a human embryonic cell with nonhuman (bovine) proteins is to be prohibited. Proteins do not encode hereditary information. The sensitivity remains in the area of mixing genomes (DNA) of human and animal, likely not the mixing of proteins, especially in the surrogate protocol under discussion wherein the bovine proteins are rapidly replaced by human.

We therefore respectfully request that Congress be measured and forward-thinking, taking into full account the tools necessary for medical researchers to apply these exciting new technologies in clinical practice in the future.

6

Embryonic Stem Cell Research Is Unethical

Center for Bioethics and Human Dignity

The Center for Bioethics and Human Dignity (CBHD) is an organization dedicated to addressing current biomedical issues such as euthanasia, reproductive technologies, and genetic intervention. The CBHD is based at Trinity International University in Bannockburn, Illinois.

Despite the existing congressional ban on federal funding for human embryo experimentation that involves the destruction of embryos, the Department of Health and Human Services (DHHS) contends that human embryonic stem (ES) cell research is legal. In addition, DHHS argues that ES cell research should be federally funded because the use of ES cells is distinct from the destruction of embryos. However, ES cells are obtained by destroying embryos, which violates the current ban. No benefits from ES research can possibly outweigh the moral cost of destroying human life. Researchers must renew their focus on alternative ways to improve medicine and relieve human suffering.

R ecent scientific advances in human stem cell research have brought into fresh focus the dignity and status of the human embryo. These advances have prompted a decision by the Department of Health and Human Services (HHS) and the National Institutes of Health (NIH) to fund stem cell research which is dependent upon the destruction of human embryos. Moreover, the National Bioethics Advisory Commission (NBAC) is calling for a modification of the current ban against federally funded human embryo research in order to permit direct federal funding for the destructive harvesting of stem cells from human embryos. These developments require that the legal, ethical, and scientific issues associated with this research be critically addressed and articulated. Our careful consideration of these issues leads to the conclusion that human stem cell research requiring the destruction of human embryos is objectionable on legal, ethical, and scientific grounds. Moreover, destruction of human embryonic life is unnecessary for medical progress, as alternative methods

Excerpted from "Human Embryos and Stem Cell Research: An Appeal for Legally and Ethically Responsible Science and Public Policy," by the Center for Bioethics and Human Dignity, www.stemcellresearch.org, August 21, 2001. Copyright © 2001 by the Center for Bioethics and Human Dignity. Reprinted with permission.

45

of obtaining human stem cells and of repairing and regenerating human tissue exist and continue to be developed. [President George W. Bush has allowed the partial federal funding of ES cell research.]

Human embryonic stem cell research violates existing law and policy

In November 1998, two independent teams of U.S. scientists reported that they had succeeded in isolating and culturing stem cells obtained from human embryos and fetuses. Stem cells are the cells from which all 210 different kinds of tissue in the human body originate. Because many diseases result from the death or dysfunction of a single cell type, scientists believe that the introduction of healthy cells of this type into a patient may restore lost or compromised function. Now that human embryonic stem cells can be isolated and multiplied in the laboratory, some scientists believe that treatments for a variety of diseases—such as diabetes, heart disease, Alzheimer's, and Parkinson's—may be within reach. While we in no way dispute the fact that the ability to treat or heal suffering persons is a great good, we also recognize that not all methods of achieving a desired good are morally or legally justifiable. If this were not so, the medically accepted and legally required practices of informed consent and of seeking to do no harm to the patient could be ignored whenever some "greater good" seems achievable.

One of the great hallmarks of American law has been its solicitous protection of the lives of individuals, especially the vulnerable. Our nation's traditional protection of human life and human rights derives from an affirmation of the essential dignity of every human being. Likewise, the international structure of human rights law—one of the great achievements of the modern world—is founded on the conviction that when the dignity of one human being is assaulted, all of us are threatened. The duty to protect human life is specifically reflected in the homicide laws of all 50 states. Furthermore, federal law and the laws of many states specifically protect vulnerable human embryos from harmful experimentation. Yet in recently publicized experiments, stem cells have been harvested from human embryos in ways which destroy the embryos.

Despite an existing congressional ban on federally-funded human embryo research, the Department of Health and Human Services (HHS) determined on January 15, 1999 that the government may fund human embryonic stem cell research. The stated rationales behind this decision are that stem cells are not embryos (which itself may be a debatable point) and that research using cells obtained by destroying human embryos can be divorced from the destruction itself. However, even NBAC denies this latter claim, as is evident by the following statement in its May 6, 1999 Draft Report on Stem Cell Research:

> Whereas researchers using fetal tissue are not responsible for the death of the fetus, researchers using stem cells derived from embryos will typically be implicated in the destruction of the embryo. This is true whether or not researchers participate in the derivation of embryonic stem cells. As long as embryos are destroyed as part of the re-

search enterprise, researchers using embryonic stem cells (and those who fund them) will be complicit in the death of embryos.

If the flawed rationales of HHS are accepted, federally-funded researchers may soon be able to experiment on stem cells obtained by destroying embryonic human beings, so long as the act of destruction does not itself receive federal funds. However, the very language of the existing ban prohibits the use of federal funds to support "research in which a human embryo or embryos are destroyed, discarded, or knowingly subjected to risk of injury or death. . . ." Obviously, Congress' intent here was not merely to prohibit the use of federal funds for embryo destruction, but to prohibit the use of such funds for research dependent in any way upon such destruction. Therefore, the opinion of HHS that human embryonic stem cell research may receive federal funding clearly violates both the language of and intention behind the existing law. Congress and the courts should ensure that the law is properly interpreted and enforced to ban federal funding for research which harms, destroys, or is dependent upon the destruction of human embryos.

Human stem cell research . . . is objectionable on legal, ethical, and scientific grounds.

It is important to recognize also that research involving human embryos outside the womb—such as embryos produced in the laboratory by in vitro fertilization (IVF) or cloning—has never received federal funding. Initially, this was because a federal regulation of 1975 prevented government funding of IVF experiments unless such experiments were deemed acceptable by an Ethics Advisory Board. Following the failure of the first advisory board to reach a consensus on the matter, no administration chose to appoint a new board. After this regulation was rescinded by Congress in 1993, the Human Embryo Research Panel recommended to the National Institutes of Health (NIH) that certain kinds of harmful nontherapeutic experiments using human embryos receive federal funding. However, these recommendations were rejected in part by former President Bill Clinton and then rejected in their entirety by Congress.

Further, it is instructive to note that the existing law which permits researchers to use fetal tissue obtained from elective abortions requires that the abortions are performed for reasons which are entirely unrelated to the research objectives. This law thus prohibits HHS from promoting the destruction of human life in the name of medical progress, yet medical progress is precisely the motivation and justification offered for the destruction of human life that occurs when stem cells are obtained from human embryos.

Current law against funding research in which human embryos are harmed and destroyed reflects well-established national and international legal and ethical norms against the misuse of any human being for research purposes. Since 1975, those norms have been applied to unborn children at every stage of development in the womb, and since 1995 they have been applied to the human embryo outside the womb as well. The existing law on human embryonic research is a reflection of universally accepted principles governing experiments on human subjects—principles reflected in the Nuremberg Code, the World Medical Association's Declaration of Helsinki, the United Nations Declaration of Human Rights, and many other statements. Accordingly, members of the human species who cannot give informed consent for research should not be the subjects of an experiment unless they personally may benefit from it or the experiment carries no significant risk of harming them. Only by upholding such research principles do we prevent treating people as things—as mere means to obtaining knowledge or benefits for others.

Public sentiment . . . seems even more opposed to government funding of embryo experimentation than to the funding of abortion.

It may strike some as surprising that legal protection of embryonic human beings can co-exist with the U.S. Supreme Court's 1973 legalization of abortion. However, the Supreme Court has never prevented the government from protecting prenatal life outside the abortion context, and public sentiment also seems even more opposed to government funding of embryo experimentation than to the funding of abortion. The laws of a number of states—including Louisiana, Maine, Massachusetts, Michigan, Minnesota, Pennsylvania, Rhode Island, and Utah—specifically protect embryonic human beings outside the womb. Most of these provisions prohibit experiments on embryos outside the womb. We believe that the above legally acknowledged protections against assaults on human dignity must be extended to all human beings—irrespective of gender, race, religion, health, disability, or age. Consequently, the human embryo must not be subject to willful destruction even if the stated motivation is to help others. Therefore, on existing legal grounds alone, research using stem cells derived from the destruction of early human embryos is proscribed.

Human embryonic stem cell research is unethical

The HHS decision and the recommendations of NBAC to federally fund research involving the destruction of human embryos would be profoundly disturbing even if this research could result in great scientific and medical gain. The prospect of government-sponsored experiments to manipulate and destroy human embryos should make us all lie awake at night. That some individuals would be destroyed in the name of medical science constitutes a threat to us all. Recent statements claiming that human embryonic stem cell research is too promising to be slowed or prohibited underscore the sort of utopianism and hubris that could blind us to the truth of what we are doing and the harm we could cause to ourselves and others. Human embryos are not mere biological tissues or clusters of cells; they are the tiniest of human beings. Thus, we have a moral responsibility not to deliberately harm them.

An international scientific consensus now recognizes that human embryos are biologically human beings beginning at fertilization and ac-knowledges the physical continuity of human growth and development from the one-cell stage forward. In the 1970s and 1980s, some frog and mouse embryologists referred to the human embryo in its first week or two of development as a "pre-embryo," claiming that it deserved less re-spect than embryos in later stages of development. However, some em-bryology textbooks now openly refer to the term "pre-embryo" as a sci-entifically invalid and "inaccurate" term which has been "discarded," and others which once used the term have quietly dropped it from new edi-tions. Both the Human Embryo Research Panel and the National Bioethics Advisory Commission have also rejected the term, describing the human embryo from its earliest stages as a living organism and a "de-veloping form of human life." The claim that an early human embryo be-comes a human being only after 14 days or implantation in the womb is therefore a scientific myth. Finally, the historic and well-respected 1995 Ramsey Colloquium statement on embryo research acknowledges that:

> The [embryo] is human; it will not articulate itself into some other kind of animal. Any being that is human is a hu-man being. If it is objected that, at five days or fifteen days, the embryo does not look like a human being, it must be pointed out that this is precisely what a human being looks like—and what each of us looked like—at five or fifteen days of development.

Therefore, the term "pre-embryo," and all that it implies, is scientifi-cally invalid.

The last century and a half has been marred by numerous atrocities against vulnerable human beings in the name of progress and medical ben-efit. In the 19th century, vulnerable human beings were bought and sold in the town square as slaves and bred as though they were animals. In the 20th century, the vulnerable were executed mercilessly and subjected to de-meaning experimentation at Dachau and Auschwitz. At mid-century, the vulnerable were subjects of our own government's radiation experiments without their knowledge or consent. Likewise, vulnerable African-Americans in Tuskegee, Alabama were victimized as subjects of a government-sponsored research project to study the effects of syphilis. Cur-rently, we are witness to the gross abuse of mental patients used as subjects in purely experimental research. These experiments were and are driven by a crass utilitarian ethos which results in the creation of a "sub-class" of hu-man beings, allowing the rights of the few to be sacrificed for the sake of potential benefit to the many. These unspeakably cruel and inherently wrong acts against human beings have resulted in the enactment of laws and policies which require the protection of human rights and liberties, in-cluding the right to be protected from the tyranny of the quest for scientific progress. The painful lessons of the past should have taught us that human beings must not be conscripted for research without their permission—no matter what the alleged justification—especially when that research means the forfeiture of their health or lives. Even if an individual's death is be-lieved to be otherwise imminent, we still do not have a license to engage in lethal experimentation—just as we may not experiment on death row pris-oners or harvest their organs without their consent.

We are aware that a number of Nobel scientists endorse human embryonic stem cell research on the basis that it may offer a great good to those who are suffering. While we acknowledge that the desire to heal people is certainly a laudable goal and understand that many have invested their lives in realizing this goal, we also recognize that we are simply not free to pursue good ends via unethical means. Of all human beings, embryos are the most defenseless against abuse. A policy promoting the use and destruction of human embryos would repeat the failures of the past. The intentional destruction of some human beings for the alleged good of other human beings is wrong. Therefore, on ethical grounds alone, research using stem cells obtained by destroying human embryos is ethically proscribed.

Human embryonic stem cell research is scientifically questionable

Integral to the decision to use federal funds for research on human embryonic stem cells is the distinction between stem cells and embryos. HHS has stated that federal funds may be used to support human embryonic stem cell research because stem cells are not embryos. A statement issued by the Office of the General Counsel of HHS regarding this decision asserts that "The statutory prohibition on the use of [government] funds . . . for human embryo research would not apply to research utilizing human pluripotent stem cells because such cells are not a human embryo within the statutory definition. [Moreover, because] pluripotent stem cells do not have the capacity to develop into a human being, [they] cannot be considered human embryos consistent with the commonly accepted or scientific understanding of that term."

The claim that an early human embryo becomes a human being only after 14 days or implantation in the womb is . . . a scientific myth.

It is important to note that the materials used in an experiment, as well as the methods of experimentation, are considered to be part of scientific research. When a scientific study is published, the first part of the article details the methods and materials used to conduct the research. Ethical and scientific evaluation of an experiment takes into account both the methods and materials used in the research process. Therefore, the source of stem cells obtained for research is both a scientifically and ethically relevant consideration.

Research on human embryonic stem cells is objectionable due to the fact that such research necessitates the prior destruction of human embryos; however, the HHS's claim that stem cells are not, and cannot develop into, embryos may itself be subject to dispute. Some evidence suggests that stem cells cultured in the laboratory may have a tendency to recongregate and form an aggregate of cells capable of beginning to develop as an embryo. In 1993, Canadian scientists reported that they successfully produced a live-born mouse from a cluster of mouse stem cells.

While it is true that these stem cells had to be wrapped in placenta-like cells in order to implant in a female mouse, it seems that at least some doubt has been cast on the claim that a cluster of stem cells is not embryonic in nature. If embryonic stem cells do indeed possess the ability to form or develop as a human embryo (without any process of activation which affects the transformation of the cell into a human embryo), research on such stem cells could itself involve the creation and/or destruction of human life and would thereby certainly fall under the existing ban on federally-funded embryo research. It would be irresponsible for the HHS to conduct and condone human embryonic stem cell research without first discerning the status of these cells. Their use in any research in which they could be converted into human embryos should likewise be banned.

Alternative to embryonic stem cell research

While proponents of human embryonic stem cell research lobby aggressively for government funding of research requiring the destruction of human embryos, alternative methods for repairing and regenerating human tissue render such an approach unnecessary for medical progress.

For instance, a promising source of more mature stem cells for the treatment of disease is hematopoietic (blood cell-producing) stem cells from bone marrow or even from the placenta or umbilical cord blood in live births. These cells are already widely used in cancer treatment and in research on treating leukemia and other diseases. Recent experiments have indicated that their versatility is even greater than once thought. For example, given the right environment, bone marrow cells can be used to regenerate muscle tissue, opening up a whole new avenue of potential therapies for muscular dystrophies. In April 1999, new advances were announced in isolating mesenchymal cells from bone marrow and directing them to form fat, cartilage, and bone tissue. Experts in stem cell research believe that these cells may allow for tissue replacement in patients suffering from cancer, osteoporosis, dental disease, or injury.

An enormously promising new source of more mature stem cells is fetal bone marrow, a source which is many times more effective than adult bone marrow and umbilical cord blood. It appears that fetal bone marrow cells do not provoke immune reactions to the same degree as adult or even newborn infant cells. This is true whether the unborn child is the donor or the recipient—that is, fetal cells can be used to treat adults, or adult bone marrow cells can be used to treat a child in the womb without the usual risk of harmful immune reactions. Such cells would not need to be derived from fetuses who were intentionally aborted, but could instead be obtained from spontaneously aborted fetuses or stillborn infants.

A policy promoting the use and destruction of human embryos would repeat the failures of the past.

In 1999, unprecedented advances were also made in isolating and culturing neural stem cells from living human nerve tissue and even from adult cadavers. Such advances render it quite possible that treatment of neural diseases such as Parkinson's and Alzheimer's, as well as spinal cord injuries, will not depend upon destructive embryo research.

Earlier claims that embryonic stem cells are uniquely capable of "self-renewal" and indefinite growth can also now be seen as premature. For example, scientists have isolated an enzyme, telomerase, which may allow human tissues to grow almost indefinitely. Although this enzyme has been linked to the development of cancer, researchers have been able to use it in a controlled way to "immortalize" useful tissue without producing cancerous growths or other harmful side effects. Thus, cultures of non-embryonic stem cells may be induced to grow and develop almost indefinitely for clinical use.

Earlier claims that embryonic stem cells are uniquely capable of "self-renewal" and indefinite growth can . . . now be seen as premature.

One of the most exciting new advances in stem cell research is the January 1999 announcement that Canadian and Italian researchers succeeded in producing new blood cells from neural stem cells taken from an adult mouse. Until recently, it was believed that adult stem cells were capable of producing only a particular type of cell: for example, a neural stem cell could develop only into cells belonging to the nervous system. Researchers believed that only embryonic stem cells retained the capacity to form all kinds of tissue in the human body. However, if stem cells taken from adult patients can produce cells and tissues capable of functioning within entirely different systems, new brain tissue needed to treat a patient with Parkinson's disease, for example, might be generated from blood stem cells derived from the patient's bone marrow. Conversely, neural stem cells might be used to produce needed blood and bone marrow. Use of a patient's own stem cells would circumvent one of the major obstacles posed by the use of embryonic stem cells—namely, the danger that tissue taken from another individual would be rejected when transplanted into a patient. Thus, in commenting on this finding, the *British Medical Journal* remarked on January 30, 1999 that the use of embryonic stem cells "may soon be eclipsed by the more readily available and less controversial adult stem cells." Given that the function of the adult stem cells was converted without the cells first having to pass through an embryonic stage, the use of such cells would not be subject to the ethical and legal objections raised by the use of human embryonic stem cells. The Director of the NIH has pointed out that evidence that adult stem cells can take on different functions has emerged only from studies on mice. However, his own claim that human embryonic stem cell research can produce treatments for diabetes and other diseases is also based solely on experimental success in mice.

One approach to tissue regeneration that does not rely on stem cells at all, but on somatic cell gene therapy, is already in use as an experimental treatment. A gene that controls production of growth factors can be injected directly into a patient's own cells, with the result that new blood vessels will develop. In early trials, this type of therapy saved the legs of patients who would have otherwise undergone amputation. It was reported in January 1999 that the technique has generated new blood vessels in the human heart and improved the condition of 19 out of 20 patients with blocked cardiac blood vessels. Such growth factors are now being explored as a means for growing new organs and tissues of many kinds.

The above recent advances suggest that it is not even necessary to obtain stem cells by destroying human embryos in order to treat disease. A growing number of researchers believe that adult stem cells may soon be used to develop treatments for afflictions such as cancer, immune disorders, orthopedic injuries, congestive heart failure, and degenerative diseases. Such researchers are working to further research on adult, rather than embryonic, stem cells. In light of these promising new scientific advances, we urge Congress to provide federal funding for the development of methods to repair and regenerate human tissue which do not require the destruction of embryonic human life. However, even if such methods do not prove to be as valuable in treating disease as are human embryonic stem cells, use of the latter in the name of medical progress is still neither legally nor ethically justifiable for the reasons stated in this document.

The utilitarian devaluation of human beings

We believe that an examination of the legal, ethical, and scientific issues associated with human embryonic stem cell research leads to the conclusion that the use of federal funds to support any such research that necessitates the destruction of human embryos is, and should remain, prohibited by law. Therefore, we call on Congress to (1) maintain the existing ban against harmful federally-funded human embryo research and make explicit its application to stem cell research requiring the destruction of human embryos and (2) provide federal funding for the development of alternative treatments which do not require the destruction of human embryonic life. If anything is to be gained from the cruel atrocities committed against human beings in the last century and a half, it is the lesson that the utilitarian devaluation of one group of human beings for the alleged benefit of others is a price we simply cannot afford to pay.

7

The Immediate Benefits of Embryonic Stem Cell Research Are Exaggerated

Charles Krauthammer

Charles Krauthammer is a syndicated columnist and contributing editor to the Weekly Standard, *a magazine of political analysis.*

Some contend that embryonic stem (ES) cell research should be urgently supported because researchers are on the brink of curing conditions such as Parkinson's disease, cancer, and spinal cord injuries. In reality, ES technology is in the elementary stage of development. Scientists have yet to fully understand the properties of stem cells and how to control them. For example, in one ES cell experiment, a human subject developed a deadly tumor as a direct result of an ES cell injection. Although stem cell research may ultimately lead to effective treatments and cures, results will not be seen for decades. The claim that restricting ES cell research denies hope to today's sick and ailing is manipulative political rhetoric.

S anity and prudence combined to produce a great victory on July 31, 2001, when the House of Representatives overwhelmingly defeated—the margin was over 100 votes—the legalization of early human embryonic cloning. But the fight is not over. The Senate needs to act as well. [It also banned embryonic cloning.]

Before it does, however, it is worth preparing oneself for the gale-force hype that Senate advocates will unleash in defense of the indefensible. One has only to look at the debate on the floor of the House to see the extraordinary lengths to which the biotech industry and its allies in Congress will go to sell the deliberate creation of embryo factories for the sole purpose of exploiting and then destroying them.

While the media have been snooping under Gary Condit's [congressman questioned in the missing person case of Chandra Levy] bed, they have missed the real scandal of the season, the unconscionable deployment of fantasy and false hopes by advocates of "therapeutic" cloning for

Excerpted from "The Great Stem Cell Hoax," by Charles Krauthammer, *The Weekly Standard*, August 20–August 27, 2001. Copyright © 2001 by *The Weekly Standard*. Reprinted with permission.

the production of stem cells. The basic premise—cure of the incurable— was stated by a *Newsweek* cover in July 2001: "There's Hope for Alzheimer's, Heart Disease, Parkinson's and Diabetes. But Will [George W.] Bush Cut Off the Money?" The theme has been echoed and reechoed nowhere more than in Congress.

The cosponsor of a permissive cloning bill, Peter Deutsch (D-FL), said this about the opposing bill totally banning cloning: "No one knows who is going to get Alzheimer's or Parkinson's or cancer. . . . What this legislation would do would be to stop the research . . . so that you could survive, so that someone who is a quadriplegic could walk, so that someone who has Alzheimer's . . ." He trailed away. You get the drift. The lion will lie down with the lamb.

Nancy Pelosi (D-CA), with characteristic subtlety: "Mr. Speaker, the National Institutes of Health and Science hold the biblical power of a cure for us."

Zoe Lofgren (D-CA): "If your religious beliefs will not let you accept a cure for your child's cancer, so be it. But do not expect the rest of America to let their loved ones suffer without cure."

Jerrold Nadler (D-NY): "We must not say to millions of sick or injured human beings, 'go ahead and die, stay paralyzed, because we believe the blastocyst, the clump of cells, is more important than you are.' . . . It is a sentence of death to millions of Americans."

Anna Eshoo (D-CA): "As we stand on the brink of finding the cures to diseases that have plagued so many millions of Americans, unfortunately, the Congress today in my view is on the brink of prohibiting this critical research."

The brink?

Eshoo gets the prize. The brink? The claim that cloning, and the stem cells it might produce, is on the verge of bringing a cure to your sick father with Alzheimer's or your debilitated mother with Parkinson's is a scandal. It is a cruel deception perpetrated by cynical scientists and ignorant politicians. Its purpose is clear: to exploit the desperation of the sick to garner political support for ethically problematic biotechnology.

The brink? Cloning animals, let alone humans, is so imperfect and difficult that it took 277 attempts before Dolly the sheep was cloned. [Dolly was cloned by embryologist Ian Wilmut and his colleagues in 1997.] Scientists estimate that the overall failure rate for cloning farm animals is 95 percent or greater. New experiments with cloned mice have shown gross deformities. And here is the worst part. We have no idea why. We understand little about how reprogrammed genes work. Scientists don't even know how to screen with any test for epigenetic abnormality.

In other words: Even if you could grow embryonic stem cells out of grandma's skin cells, we have no idea yet how to regulate and control these cells in a way to effect a cure. Just growing them in tissue culture is difficult enough. Then you have to tweak them to make precisely the kind of cells grandma needs. Then you have to inject them and hope to God that you don't kill her.

We have already had one such experience, a human stem cell experiment in China. Embryonic stem cells were injected into a suffering Parkinson's patient. The results were horrific. Because we don't yet know how to control stem cells, they grew wildly and developed into one of the most primitive and terrifying cancers, a "teratoma." When finally autopsied—the cure killed the poor soul—they found at the brain site of the injection a tumor full of hair, bone and skin.

Let's have a little honesty in both the cloning and stem cell debates. Stem cell research does hold promise for clinical cures in the far future. But right now we're at the stage of basic science: We don't understand how these cells work, and we don't know how to control them. Because their power is so extraordinary, they are very dangerous. Elementary considerations of safety make the prospect of real clinical application distant.

For future generations

Stem cells are the cure of the mid 21st century. Stem cell research deserves support because the basic research needs to be done and we might as well get started now. But the cure is for future generations. The cynical appeal to curing grandma is raw exploitation of misery. Nothing of the sort is about to happen. Those who claim it ought to be ashamed.

But rather than exhibit shame, the scientific community is rallying—in the name of retaining their autonomy from the ignorant dictates of lay society—to sugarcoat the news. Most notorious is the case of the research article on embryonic stem cells published in July 2001 in the journal *Science*, one of the most respected scientific publications in the world. The research showed that embryonic stem cells of mice are genetically unstable. Yes, you can make them grow over and over again, but we don't know how or why some genes are turned on and off. You can make a million copies of a stem cell. They may be genetically identical. But if different genes are turned on in the various cells, the results—the properties of the tissue or organism they develop into—can be wildly different.

Even if you could grow embryonic stem cells out of grandma's skin cells, we have no idea yet how to regulate and control these cells.

Now the really bad news. The authors of that study initially had a sentence at the end of the paper stating the obvious conclusion that this research might put in question the clinical applicability of stem cell research.

But that cannot be said publicly. In a highly unusual move, the authors withdrew the phrase that the genetic instability of stem cells "might limit their use in clinical applications" just a few days before publication. They instead emphasized that this mouse study ought not hold back stem cell research.

This change in text represents a corruption of science that mirrors the corruption of language in the congressional debate. It is corrupting because this study might have helped to undermine the extravagant claims made by stem cell advocates that a cure for Parkinson's or spinal cord injury or Alzheimer's is in the laboratory and just around the corner, if only those right-wing, antiabortion nuts would let it go forward.

In reviewing a book on Parkinson's disease, Nina King, associate editor of *Washington Post Book World*, noted that when she was diagnosed with the disease 15 years ago, she was told that a cure was 5 or 10 years away. She has heard that ever since. A cure in 5 to 10 years "is like a mirage on the horizon, glowing with promise but ever receding."

The march of science

The other scandalous myth being perpetrated, besides imminence, is inevitability. It goes like this:

The march of science will go on. Legislators can try to contain the growth of knowledge, but it is futile. Somebody somewhere will work on stem cells or cloning. So let us at least take it out of the closet and keep it in the public eye.

What this mantra does not take into account is the radical effect a ban on anything in science has on the quality and quantity of people working on it. Cloning has not even been banned, but because it is societally disapproved of, it is generally shunned by serious researchers. Look at the cloning conference called by the National Academy of Sciences on August 7, 2001, in Washington. [Cloning for any purpose was banned in the United States in 2001.] A vast majority of researchers there view with horror the cloning of a human child—except for three researchers who declared their determination to do it. Three in the whole world.

One looked less stable than the other. Dr. Brigitte Boisselier recently closed her "Clonaid" laboratory in the United States and is supposedly opening one offshore. When she spoke to the gathered about the right to do what one wants with one's genes, she did not inspire great confidence, possibly because she is a member of the Raelian sect, a cult founded by a former French race car driver after being visited by aliens in 1973. Seeing how marginalized cloning researchers [were] even before a legal ban, one can imagine how much more marginalized they will be after one.

A ban works by robbing outlawed research of the best and the brightest. They are not going to devote their lives to a career where they must work in the shadows, ostracized, and under threat of arrest. That ought to encourage legislators to believe that society can indeed influence the direction of science.

Yes, in the very long run some science will break through. But one must not underestimate the efficacy of political restraint. If you can restrain for decades something that promises a cure, imagine how many other, less morally repulsive, substitute cures will present themselves in the meantime. You cannot stop evil science, but you can delay it, and thus possibly supplant it.

That is why the House action banning all cloning was so important. The Senate must demonstrate its seriousness, too. Now that the president has permitted only research from existing stem cell lines, the Democratic Senate is sure to try to loosen that standard and permit stem cell research from discarded fertility clinic embryos as well. But until Congress has demonstrated its seriousness about preventing the creation of embryo factories for exploitation by banning cloning completely, it cannot be trusted on any question regarding human manufacture.

8

Early Human Embryos Are Human Beings

Andrew Sullivan

Andrew Sullivan is an independent journalist and author of Virtually Normal: An Argument About Homosexuality.

Arguments that early human embryos—which are destroyed during embryonic stem cell (ES) research—are not human beings and can be subjected to experimentation are flawed. First, the claim that early human embryos, or blastocysts, are not human beings because they cannot live outside the womb or without medical help leads inevitably to the conclusion that adults who are on life support are not human either. Second, arguments that blastocysts are not human beings because they lack sentience opens the door to experimentation upon adult human beings with Alzheimer's or other debilitating diseases. Ultimately, blastocysts deserve all the rights of human beings, especially the right to respect and dignity.

In one of the creepiest scenarios in Steven Spielberg and Stanley Kubrick's new movie *A.I.*, there is something called a Flesh Fair. In this sci-fi fantasy, human beings have developed technology so refined that they can create mechanical humans that appear almost as real as organic ones. These "mechas" are essentially a slave class: They perform chores, replace lost children, even have their body parts distributed for various uses. At Flesh Fairs, mechas are displayed and killed for amusement, their body parts sometimes traded and reused. They are humans entirely as means—not ends. And, of course, they're not truly human at all. They're robots simulating humans. But even robots, Spielberg and Kubrick seem to suggest, merit some dignity.

If robots deserve dignity, shouldn't blastocysts [early human embryos]? In thinking about stem-cell research, the image of the Flesh Fair still resonates. In *A.I.* humans use pseudo-humans for sport; they chop them up, dissect them, then throw them away. When we watch the movie, we naturally recoil. But when we read essentially the same story in the newspapers—about events happening now—we manage to keep calm.

Excerpted from "Only Human," by Andrew Sullivan, *The New Republic*, July 30, 2001. Copyright © 2001 by The New Republic, Inc. Reprinted with permission.

Is the analogy a stretch? Supporters of stem-cell research say blastocysts are not human beings. Or, even if they are human, they are not beings. They are no more human than, say, a clipped fingernail (which contains all the DNA information for an entire person, just as accurately as a blastocyst). Clearly, however, the fingernail comparison misses something important. A fingernail would not become a mature human being if implanted in a womb. The real question is whether this distinction amounts to a moral difference.

Equal grist for the scientific mill

One criterion to distinguish a real human being—with rights and dignity—from an embryo or a fingernail might be viability. The blastocyst, while clearly the same species as the rest of us, cannot survive independent of scientific paraphernalia, a freezer, or a womb. Hence it's not a human being—and can morally be experimented on. That's a clear line—but it opens up a host of other possibilities. If "viability" independent of a mother or others is the criterion, why shouldn't the physically incapacitated or the very old be consigned to medical experimentation? Why not those in comas or on life support? If they're going to die anyway and have no ability to fend for themselves, what's the point of wasting their bodies when they could yield valuable medical insights? Yes, we could wait till they're dead—but they're far more useful to science alive.

A blastocyst is the purest form of human being.

Other criteria might be the ability to feel pain, think rationally, or be self-conscious. Since an embryo (so far as we know) can do none of these things, it's fair game. But again, these criteria make others who are similarly limited—such as those with Alzheimer's, or the paraplegic, or the insane—equal grist for the scientific mill. This is especially the case with those whose mental capacity renders them unable to give meaningful consent. Why ask at all if, like embryos, such pseudo-humans cannot say yes or no? Perhaps some people might even give their consent in advance for such work. For ethical purposes, these people could be protected from physical pain during experimentation until their death.

Defining a "human being"

Supporters of stem-cell research won't go that far. Except that they already have. What, after all, makes a human being a human being? Scientists would say a human is defined by its DNA—the genetic coding that makes our species different from any others. Stem-cell research enthusiasts say we are defined by our DNA *and* our stage of development. They say a blastocyst is so unformed that it cannot be equated with a fetus, let alone with an adult. But it remains a fact—indeed one of the marvels of creation—that the embryo contains exactly the same amount of genetic information as you or I do. We aren't different from it in kind, only different in degree: in age, size, weight, gender, and on and on. In fact, in some sense, a blastocyst is the purest form of human being—genderless, indistinguishable to the naked eye from any other, unencumbered with the accoutrements of society and experience—and yet as unique as any human being who has ever lived or ever will. To extinguish it is surely not to extinguish something other than us. It is to extinguish us.

Consider these analogies. Federal law makes it a crime to kill or injure a bald eagle. It is also a crime to kill or injure a bald eagle's egg. We recognize that to kill one is the same as to kill the other. Similarly, I cannot remember the last time an apple farmer responded to an early frost by saying, "Never mind, we lost the fertilized blossom, but the apples will be fine." Of course, the apples won't be fine. Once the blossom is dead, the apples will never arrive. And once a blastocyst is killed, the human being coiled inexorably inside is no more. If that isn't killing, what is? And why are we more coherent when it comes to eagles than when it comes to humans?

Treating human life instrumentally

Some may say that nature itself allows many blastocysts to die. What else are miscarriages? It is true that such tragedies happen all the time. But just because earthquakes happen doesn't mean massacres are justified. And our intuitive moral response to a woman who has had a miscarriage is not the same as our response to a woman who has had a haircut or even to a woman who has lost a limb. One might conceivably justify allowing extra blastocysts to be created and lost as collateral damage in an artificial insemination (although, the more I think about this, the less defensible it seems). But to turn around and use those extra blastocysts for experimentation is a completely separate step. It is to treat human life purely instrumentally. I know of no better description of evil.

Such evil cannot be morally counterbalanced by any good that medical breakthroughs might bring. This is especially true when it's possible to cultivate stem cells from other sources. Perhaps those sources are not as fecund as embryos—but that means we are confronted not by a trade-off between *any* research into stem cells and preserving human life, but between better, faster stem-cell research and human life. Under those conditions, it's not that close a call. After all, are we currently beset by the problem of scientific breakthroughs that aren't fast enough? Surely the opposite is true (or at least *also* true): We are beset by scientific break-throughs that are occurring far faster than we have the moral language or the experience to deal with. Is a slight deceleration in that research too high a price to pay for removing even the chance that we may be taking human life?

I'm not dismissing the real pain of those dying of terminal illnesses who might conceivably be saved by this research—or the pain of their families. We should indeed do all we can to end and abate any and all disease. I write as someone with a deeply vested interest in such research. But life should be measured not by how long it is lived but by how it is lived. If my life were extended one day at the expense of one other human's life itself, it would be an evil beyond measure. Some things cannot be simply bargained or rationalized away. And one of those things is surely life itself.

9

Cloning Human Embryos for Therapeutic Purposes Should Be Banned

Mae-Wan Ho and Joe Cummins

Mae-Wan Ho is founder and director of the Institute of Science in Society (I-SIS), a nonprofit organization based in London, England, that seeks to maintain social responsibility within the fields of scientific research and application. Joe Cummins is professor emeritus of genetics at the University of West Ontario in London, Ontario, Canada.

Many argue that cloning human embryos will benefit medical science because embryonic stem (ES) cells may give rise to—and potentially replace—almost all types of human tissue when they degenerate. However, creating and destroying human embryos for scientific and medical purposes is morally unacceptable because it involves the destruction of life. In addition, it opens the door to the unethical practices of reproductive cloning and eugenics. The rush to advance ES cell and cloning technologies is driven by the commercial interests of powerful biotechnical companies, not by concerns for human health.

What are stem cells?

Stems cells are cells in mammals including human beings that have the ability to divide and give rise to specialized, differentiated cells. The fertilized egg cell possesses this ability to the highest degree, for it has the potential to divide and develop into the entire organism with the full complement of cell types. The fertilized egg cell is *totipotent*.

Totipotency is retained as the egg divides into two and even four cells, so that each cell, when separated, is capable of developing into a complete foetus. That is how twins, triplets and quadruplets come about; they are natural human clones with identical genetic *and* cytoplasmic makeup.

When the embryo is four days old, and after several rounds of cell division, a hollow sphere is formed, called a *blastocyst*, within which is a cluster of cells called the *inner cell mass*. The outer layer is destined to

Excerpted from "The Unnecessary Evil of 'Therapeutic' Human Cloning," by Mae-Wan Ho and Joe Cummins, *Institute of Science in Society Report*, January 23, 2001. Copyright © 2001 by The Institute of Science in Society, www.i-sis.org. Reprinted with permission.

form the placenta and other supporting tissues needed for the development of the foetus in the womb. The inner cell mass will go on to become all the tissues of the foetus' body. These cells are no longer totipotent, but *pluripotent*, ie, they can give rise to many types of cells, but not all of the ones required for foetal development.

As development proceeds, the inner cell mass divides further and become more restricted in the range of cells they will become. For example, blood stem cells will eventually give rise to red blood cells, white blood cells and platelets, and skin stem cells will give rise to all the various types of skin cells. These more specialized stem cells are said to be *multipotent*.

Embryonic stem cells carry health risks, and there are major technical difficulties in creating them with . . . cloning techniques.

Pluripotent and multipotent stem cells in the embryo came to be known as *embryonic stem cells* or ES cells.

Stem cells are also found in children and adults; these are known as *adult stem cells*. Blood stem cells, for example, are found in the bone marrow of every child and adult, and in very small numbers, also in the blood stream; they continually replace the supply of blood cells throughout life. Recently, adult stem cells have also been found in brain as well as muscle, liver, skin and other tissues.

One of the main arguments used in favour of 'therapeutic' human embryo cloning is that adult stem cells are much more restricted in their potential to become different cell types than ES cells. However, it is beginning to appear that adult stem cells have the potential to give rise to a far greater range of cell types than previously imagined, and stunning results have been obtained. Furthermore, there are ways to obtain ES cells other than human cloning.

Embryonic stem cells are not all equal

There are three kinds of ES cells. The first is derived from the inner cell mass, a procedure pioneered in Dr. James Thomson's laboratory in the University of Wisconsin using 'excess' embryos from *in vitro* fertilization clinics. The second, embryonic germ cells, is isolated from the regions of the embryo destined to become ovaries or testes. This was first carried out by Dr. John Gearhart's group in Johns Hopkins University, using foetuses from terminated pregnancies. The cells resulting from the two laboratories appear to be very similar.

The third kind of ES cells involves somatic cell nuclear transfer, the technique that created Dolly, the lamb cloned from a cell of an adult sheep. [Dolly was cloned by embryologist Ian Wilmut and his colleagues in 1997.] Researchers take a normal human (or animal) unfertilised egg and remove the nucleus, replacing it with the nucleus from a somatic cell of a human donor. The perceived advantage of this procedure is that the somatic cell donor could be the patient requiring tissue replacement, thus avoiding problems associated with immune rejection of transplanted cells or tissues that are foreign to the body.

As is clear from the description, the first two categories of ES cells do not involve the creation of human embryos, and research on those ES cells has already been going on for the past two years. Many people may find research on those stem cells morally acceptable, though it will be difficult to justify research on those cells in view of the latest discoveries on the enormous developmental potentials of adult cells (see below), which make ES cells completely redundant.

It is research on ES cells obtained by nuclear transfer that raises the most serious moral concerns, for it requires the creation of embryos specifically for providing ES cells, the embryos being destroyed in the process.

In December 1998, researchers in the Infertility Clinic at Kyeonghee University in Korea announced that they had successfully cloned a human embryo by transferring the nucleus from the somatic cell of a 30 year old woman into one of her unfertilized eggs. This embryo was reported to have developed to the fourth cell division stage, when it would have been implanted. But it was destroyed on ethical considerations. Meanwhile, researchers in the United States and Australia have created 'human' embryos by transferring the nucleus of human cells into the eggs of the cow and the pig. It is of course questionable whether the embryos created by such procedures are human, and whether they are justifiable on moral grounds. These were destroyed at day 14. It was not clear, however, whether ES cells have been extracted from the embryos before they were destroyed.

"Therapeutic" human cloning is a slippery slope to reproductive cloning and the re-emergence of eugenics.

Proponents claim that one of the major advantages of ES cells is that established cell lines can be obtained only from ES cells and not adult stem cells; though this may no longer be true (see below).

ES cells carry health risks, and there are major technical difficulties in creating them with nuclear transplant cloning techniques.

- ES cells can give rise to teratomas—malignant tumours (cancers) consisting of a disorganized mass of differentiated cells—on being transplanted.
- Nuclear transplant cloning is a very inefficient process with massive failure rates, requiring a large number of donor eggs.
- Nuclear transplant clones created by transferring human nuclei into cow and pig eggs carry even greater risks, as it is well-known that such interspecific nuclear-cytoplasmic hybrids fail to develop normally.

Commercial interests, not public good

There are powerful commercial interests in ES stem cells. Geron Corporation of Menlo Park, California, gained first rights to exploit cells commercially, and also funded the isolation of embryonic germ cells. A total of ten companies were involved in exploiting stem cell technology and stem cells in 2000. Geron already owns dozens of patents on ES cells.

Companies investing in adult stem cell technology include Nexell Therapeutics of Irvine, California, and Anastrom Biosciences of Ann Arbor, Michigan. Osiris Therapeutics of Baltimore, Maryland, identified mesenchyme stem in the supportive tissue that surrounds the bone marrow, and has patented systems for isolating and producing those cells, and launched two clinical trials. Mesenchyme cells can differentiate into cartilage, muscle and even neurons. Neural stem cells came on the scene later, but already clinical trials have begun.

It is morally unacceptable to create human embryos for providing embryonic stem cells.

It is clear that the major impetus for both ES and adult stem cell research is coming from the biotech companies and scientists working with them. Therapy is likely to be very costly on account of the multiple license fees that have to be paid, not only on cells and cell lines but on isolation procedures.

Public opposition to 'therapeutic' human embryo cloning has been fierce. Apart from the moral objection to the creation of human embryos that are destined to be destroyed, many groups feel that 'therapeutic' human cloning is a slippery slope to reproductive cloning and the re-emergence of eugenics. The Bill Clinton administration had forbidden such research in federally funded projects; and no European Government, with the exception of the United Kingdom, is in favour of such research.

The British government first announced plans to relax the law on human embryo cloning to allow the creation of human embryos up to 14 days to provide ES cells. Parliament voted in favour of the new law in December 2000, against the advice of the European Group of Ethics in Science and New Technologies (EGE). The House of Lords endorsed Parliament's decision with an overwhelming majority January 22, 2001.

The EGE had warned that the creation of embryos by somatic cell nuclear transfer ('therapeutic cloning') for research on stem cell therapy would be premature", drawing attention to the rapidly developing research in adult stem cells. The EGE recommended that the EU should set up a budget to explore non-cloning sources of stem cells, especially adult tissue, and to enable the results of such research to be "widely disseminated."

Promises of adult stem cells

Mammals appear to contain some 20 major types of somatic stem cells. Stem cells have been described that can generate all the cells in the brain, the liver, pancreas, bone and cartilage. These adult stem cells are increasingly found to have the potential to become practically as many different cell types as ES cells. Furthermore, it appears that differentiated adult cells can be made to revert to cells remarkably similar to stem cells, and to have the ability to multiply for long periods in cell culture. Some of the findings are highlighted below.

- Mouse bone marrow stem cells can give rise to skeletal muscle and brain cells. Liver /pancreas stem cells can give rise to blood cells and brain cells. Brain cells can give rise to all previous cell types including the peripheral nervous system and smooth muscle. Brain cells have been found to differentiate to muscle, blood, intestine, liver and heart.

- Catherine Verfaillie of the University of Minnesota in Minneapolis is reported to have isolated bone marrow cells from children and adults that can become brain, liver, and muscle cells as well. These were found in adults between 45 and 50 years old. This research has not yet appeared in print.
- Scientists from the National Neurological Institute and Stem Cell Research Institute in Milan, Italy, succeeded in growing skeletal muscle from stem cells originating from an adult brain, both in culture and in animals receiving the transplanted stem cells (Galli, R. et al (2000) *Nature Neuroscience* 3, 986-991).
- A researcher in Britain, Dr. Ilham Abuljadaye, has just announced an efficient method for creating large quantities of adult stem cells from white blood cells, and her findings have been independently replicated, though not yet published. The method involves inducing the white blood cells to de-differentiate in the test-tube into stem cells ("Stem cell discovery reverses time" *The Times*, 15 Jan 2001). That means it will be feasible to prepare stem cells from the patient who is in need of cell or tissue transplant, greatly simplifying the procedure, avoiding immune reactions and reducing cost.
- Two research teams at University College London found that adult rat cells can be made to divide hundreds of times when provided with the right mixture of nutrients, and without taking on the undesirable characteristics of cancer cells, such as uncontrollable growth (Cohen, P. (2001). *New Scientist* 18 Jan). Adult human cells may have the same capacity.
- Another possibility is that the patient's own stem cells could be stimulated to multiply and replace cells and tissues within the body itself (McKay, R. (2000). *Nature* 406, 361-364.)

Unnecessary and unacceptable

We reject research on ES cells created by human 'therapeutic' cloning on the following grounds.

- It is totally unnecessary, given the promise of adult stem cells and adult cells from the patients themselves, which can be most effectively used for cell and tissue replacement.
- It is morally unacceptable to create human embryos for providing ES cells.
- It is a slippery slope to human reproductive cloning.
- Nuclear transplant cloning has very low success rates and generates many abnormalities.
- Cloning procedures involving transplanting human nuclei into animal eggs carry even greater risks.
- ES cells are already available using 'excess' embryos from *in vitro* fertilization clinics and aborted fetuses.
- ES cells carry cancer risks on being transplanted.
- ES cells are subject to multiple patents, on cloning and isolation

procedures as well as on the cells themselves; this will make their use in cell or tissue replacement therapy very costly.
- Adult stem cells are already showing great promise in cell and tissue replacement; and are likely to be much less costly.

'Therapeutic' human cloning is an unnecessary evil. We call on the United Kingdom (UK) Government to reject it in line with the other European Union (EU) countries, and to support research into non-cloning sources of stem cells, especially adult cells, with special emphasis on methods that do not involve patented procedures and cell lines.

10

Frozen Embryo Adoption Should Be Encouraged

JoAnn L. Davidson

JoAnn L. Davidson is program director for the Snowflakes Embryo Adoption Program, a division of Nightlight Christian Adoptions. The program promotes the adoption of frozen embryos as an alternative to donating them to scientific research.

In vitro fertilization is a fertility treatment in which a couple's egg and sperm are fertilized outside the womb and implanted into the woman as an embryo. Because fertility treatments produce more embryos than can be safely implanted into a womb, unused embryos are frozen so that they may be stored and used in the future. As a result, the number of frozen embryos warehoused in fertility clinics has skyrocketed. Rather than discarding or donating them to destructive embryonic research, genetic parents should have the opportunity to place their frozen embryos up for adoption. Each human embryo has the potential to become a unique individual and deserves a chance to be born.

The first development to influence Nightlight's [Christian adoption] decision was a British law passed on August 1, 1991, requiring the destruction of all frozen embryos unclaimed after five years. It took effect on July 31, 1996, leading to the extermination, according to a survey by Britain's Human Fertilization & Embryology Authority, of 3,300 frozen embryos. The genetic parents of the remaining 6,000 embryos exercised their rights to extend storage for another five years or donate them. Nightlight decided it wanted to do its part to prevent a similar massacre in the United States.

The second development is the rapid growth since the early-1980s of the in-vitro fertilization ("IVF") industry in the United States. In the last two decades, it grew from one clinic to 360 by 1998. In the late-1990s, it was estimated that the IVF industry was earning revenues exceeding $350 million annually. One observer estimated in 1999 that these IVF clinics store more than 150,000 frozen live humans with 19,000 added each

Excerpted from JoAnn L. Davidson's testimony before the House of Representatives Committee on Reform, Subcommittee on Criminal Justice, Drug Policy, and Human Resources Hearing on Embryonic Cell Research. July 17, 2001.

year. Anecdotal evidence suggests the number may be much higher.

Due to the tendency of fertility drugs given to women in IVF programs to produce more embryos than can safely be implanted at any one time, it has become common to freeze the unused embryos in a process called cryopreservation in order to preserve their lives for implantation at a later date. Although this process relieves the woman of the cost and physical burden of further egg retrievals while preserving the lives of some of their embryos, the practical result is that the IVF industry regularly produces more human embryos than it implants, leading to an exploding frozen living human population.

An increasing number of genetic parents presented with the dilemma of what to do with their frozen embryos would like the alternative of placing them with qualified families.

IVF clinics agree to store frozen embryos for a fixed period of time, usually five years. Then, they offer the genetic parents the option of extending storage for a fee varying between $100 and $500 annually, implanting the embryos, terminating them, or donating them for some purpose. Storage agreements with IVF clinics may include a presumption in favor of one of these alternatives if the genetic parents fail to act.

An increasing number of genetic parents presented with the dilemma of what to do with their frozen embryos would like the alternative of placing them with qualified families. Regardless of the medical or legal status of their embryos, these genetic parents are emotionally invested in their offspring and feel responsible for their welfare. As their storage contracts come up for renewal, they are looking for additional choices not offered by IVF clinics.

Embryo adoption

Fortunately, there are tremendous potential benefits of embryo adoption for infertile families. An estimated 6.5 to 10 million couples (or 13 to 20 million individuals) in the United States suffer from infertility. Most of them dearly want children and long to conceive. Accordingly, many turn to the IVF industry, notwithstanding the expense, the low success rate, and their ethical reservations. For these people, child adoption is less attractive, because it does not involve pregnancy, prenatal bonding, or childbirth.

In contrast, embryo adoption involves all of these benefits, includes the satisfaction of parenting a waiting child, and is far less expensive than IVF treatments. The average expense of our embryo adoptions is between $7,000 and $10,000, compared to an average of nearly $50,000 for IVF treatments plus expensive medication. Half of the couples that have participated in embryo adoption through the Snowflakes Program have become pregnant.

Embryo adoption is better than embryo donation because it involves a thorough screening process designed to ensure that embryos are placed with stable families meeting the expectations of genetic parents. It also protects against parenting paternally related children. Genetic parents complete an inventory of their financial, religious, educational and other preferences. We match these with input from the adopting parents.

Adoptive families participate in a standard home study, which can be used either for embryo or traditional adoption. They must also divulge thorough medical, psychological, paternal, and background information. The adoption agency preparing the homestudy provides professional counseling and education to the adoptive family regarding integrating the child into the home, parenting, and other issues unique to the family.

The Snowflakes Program promotes open adoption over closed adoption, because it is the most psychologically rewarding for all concerned. Open adoption necessarily involves selection of families through pictures and letters and usually, but not necessarily, involves knowledge by the genetic and adoptive parents of one another's last names and addresses. We recommend the latter because it enables children to become acquainted with their genetic parents and receive answers to the questions they naturally ask.

When we find a match between genetic and adoptive parents, we begin the formal adoption process, including drafting an adoption agreement. The latter provides, among other things, for the relinquishment of the genetic parents' rights over the embryo and states that the baby born will bear the name of the adoptive family and have inheritance rights through only the adoptive family.

Every human embryo . . . deserves to be nurtured and given a chance for a good life with an adoptive couple.

Under well-established contract law principles, embryo adoption through an adoption agreement is permitted in all 50 states. Accordingly, the fact that the legal framework for embryo adoption is partially articulated in not more than a few states is less of a concern. The presumed mother of a child is his or her birth mother, who in this case is also the adoptive mother.

Following adoption, Snowflakes arranges for shipment of the frozen living humans. Then, implantation proceeds. The adoptive family selects his or her own embryologist and other physicians who prepare the adopting woman's womb (which normally involves injections of inexpensive hormones such as estrogen and progesterone), thaw the embryos, and perform the transfer. The adoption agreement requires that any unused embryos be returned to their genetic parents. They may not be destroyed.

To date, the Snowflakes Program has been involved in the placement of eight babies born to six families across the United States. . . . Five children are in gestation in the wombs of three moms. Twenty-seven families have been matched. A total of 314 embryos from 35 families have been adopted, 182 thawed, and 93 survived and implanted.

The Snowflakes Program only recently received publicity when ABC's *PrimeTime* featured it on April 12, 2001. After the program aired, the number of genetic parents that enrolled their frozen children in the Program increased 35 percent to roughly 67 with an average of seven embryos each in storage. The number of registered adoptive families also increased to roughly 70. Recently, we learned about a group of IVF practitioners considering disbanding, who would like to offer to each of their 500 clients the adoption option.

Not in excess of the clinical need

The potential growth of the Snowflakes Program is mind-numbing. We have doubled in size each year since the program started. This past year (2000), we increased our embryo adoptions 600 percent. We are scrambling now to develop a model, which other agencies can implement, to expand the embryo adoption concept.

Ultimately, no embryo will prove in "excess of the clinical need." Based upon our conservative estimate of 188,000 frozen human embryos currently stored in IVF clinics, a conservative thaw survival rate of 50 percent, and a national pregnancy rate for IVF clinics of between 13.4% (over 40) to 37.2% (under 35), between 12,600 and 35,000 children could be placed for adoption and born in the families of the 6.5 to 10 million infertile married couples in America who seek to raise children.

Human embryo adoption is not about . . . hindering medical science, which has not exhausted potential advances with adult, placenta, and umbilical stem cells.

Every human embryo, even if he or she can no longer be cared for by their genetic parents, deserves to be nurtured and given a chance for a good life with an adoptive couple who will love and raise them to be welcome citizens of this country. Under these circumstances, a decision to authorize the federal funding of human embryo destruction is a decision to take the lives of at least 12,600 to 35,000 children who otherwise could have been born and raised by loving adoptive parents.

Therefore, independent of the legal question whether an embryo is or is not a "legal person" for this or another purpose, we respectfully request, along with most Americans (especially infertile Americans), that Congress not lift its existing ban against federal spending for the destruction of human embryos for any purpose, including the lethal "harvesting" and medical experimentation upon the stem cells that compose each living human embryo. [The ban is currently enforced.]

Poll data educating Americans on the necessary consequence of embryo stem cell research, in particular, the destruction of embryos required to obtain their stem cells, reveals that 74 percent of Americans oppose use of tax dollars to support it. The media, nevertheless, has tried to paint opposition to embryo stem cell research as another attempt to overturn *Roe v. Wade*. [This 1973 Supreme Court case led to the federal protection of the right to have an abortion.]

This is unreasonable. At least fifteen states (including Utah) have expressed their legislative intent to outlaw harmful experiments on human embryos, regardless of how they are funded. Thirty-seven states and the District of Columbia enforce tort, criminal and other laws declaring that human life begins at conception. These laws have not affected the constitutionality of the pro-choice position. Likewise, a decision to fund or not to fund embryo stem cell research has no bearing on whether a mother has the right to terminate her pregnancy.

Genocide as medical therapy

Human embryo adoption is not about abortion. It is not about hindering medical science, which has not exhausted potential advances with adult, placenta, and umbilical stem cells. It is not about "dots on a paper," as Sen. Tom Harkin has referred to living human embryos, nor like "shooting gold fish in a barrel," as actress Mary Tyler Moore likened killing living human embryos. Sad to say, this is not even about banning privately funded destructive research on living human embryos to harvest their stem cells.

Rather, this debate is about whether we as an entire society want to federally fund research destroying any chance that 6.5 to 10 million infertile couples may adopt and conceive children. Here in this room and in homes across America, we must decide whether we should compel every taxpayer to support destroying human beings at a stage of development through which each one of us passed. We have never before done this. We do not now even federally fund abortion.

In the final analysis, we must decide whether we should accept the effect of genocide, if any, as medical therapy. Having looked into the eyes of eight precious newborns and former frozen embryos, I for one will not. Instead, I urge Congress to provide more funding for the continuing research involving adult, placenta, and umbilical human stem cells to find rapid cures for life-threatening diseases.

Organizations to Contact

The editors have compiled the following list of organizations concerned with the issues debated in this book. The descriptions are derived from materials provided by the organizations. All have publications or information available for interested readers. The list was compiled on the date of publication of the present volume; the information provided here may change. Be aware that many organizations take several weeks or longer to respond to inquiries, so allow as much time as possible.

American Life League (ALL)
PO Box 1350, Stafford, VA 22555
(540) 659-4171
website: www.all.org

ALL promotes family values and opposes abortion, human embryo experimentation, and fetal organ donation. The organization monitors congressional activities dealing with pro-life issues. It produces educational materials, books, flyers, and programs for pro-family organizations. Publications include the newsletter *Communiqué* and the magazine *Celebrate Life*.

BC Biotechnology Alliance (BCBA)
3250 East Mall, Suite 220, Vancouver, BC, V6T 1W5, CANADA
(604) 221-3026 • fax: (604) 221-3027
website: www.biotech.bc.ca

The BCBA is an association for producers and users of biotechnology. The alliance works to increase public awareness and understanding of biotechnology, including the awareness of its potential contributions to society. The alliance's publications include the bimonthly newsletter *Biofax* and the annual magazine *Biotechnology in BC*.

Center for Bioethics
University of Minnesota
Suite N504 Boynton, 410 Church St. SE, Minneapolis, MN 55455
(612) 624-9440 • fax: (612) 624-9108
e-mail: bioethx@tc.umn.edu • website: www.bioethics.umn.edu

The Center for Bioethics seeks to advance and disseminate knowledge concerning ethical issues in health care and the life sciences. It conducts original research, offers educational programs, fosters public discussion and debate, and assists in the formulation of public policy. The center publishes the quarterly newsletter *Bioethics Examiner* and reading packets on specific topics, including fetal tissue experimentation.

Do No Harm: The Coalition of Americans for Research Ethics
200 Daingerfield Rd., Suite 100, Alexandria, VA 22314
(703) 684-8352 • fax: (703) 684-5813
website: www.stemcellresearch.org

Do No Harm: The Coalition of Americans for Research Ethics is a national coalition of researchers, health care professionals, bioethicists, legal professionals, and others dedicated to the promotion of scientific research and health care which does no harm to human life. The coalition opposes human embryo experimentation and research. Its website provides numerous publications, public and congressional testimonies, and commentaries on stem cell research.

The Hastings Center
Garrison, NY 10524-5555
(914) 424-4040 • fax: (914) 424-4545
e-mail: mail@thehastingscenter.org • website: www.thehastingscenter.org

Since it was founded in 1969, the Hastings Center has played a central role in responding to the ethical questions raised by advances in medicine and biotechnology. It conducts research on such issues and provides consultations. The center publishes books, papers, guidelines, and the bimonthly *Hastings Center Report*.

Human Cloning Foundation (HFC)
PMB 143, 1100 Hammond Dr., Suite 410A, Atlanta, GA 30328
website: www.humancloning.org

The foundation is a nonprofit organization that promotes the positive aspects of human cloning and related technologies, such as human embryo experimentation. The HFC's website contains numerous articles and fact sheets on the benefits of human cloning.

National Bioethics Advisory Commission (NBAC)
6100 Executive Blvd., Suite 5B01, Rockville, MD 20592-7508
(301) 402-4242 • fax: (301) 480-6900
website: www.bioethics.gov

The NBAC is a federal agency that sets guidelines to govern the ethical conduct of biotechnological research. It works to protect the rights and welfare of human research subjects and oversees the management and use of genetic information. Its published reports include *Cloning Human Beings* and *Ethical Issues in Human Stem Cell Research*.

National Right to Life Committee (NRLC)
419 Seventh St. NW, Suite 500, Washington, DC 20004
(202) 626-8800
e-mail: NRLC@nrlc.org • website: www.nrlc.org

The NRLC is one of the largest organizations opposing abortion and human embryo experimentation. The committee campaigns against legislation to legalize abortion. It encourages ratification of a constitutional amendment granting embryos and fetuses the same right to life as living persons, and it advocates alternatives to abortion and human embryo experimentation. The NRLC publishes the brochure *When Does Life Begin?* and the periodical *National Right to Life News*.

Snowflakes Embryo Adoption Program
Nightlight Christian Adoptions
801 East Chapman, Suite 106, Fullerton, CA 92831
(714) 278-1020 • fax: (714) 278-1063
e-mail: info@snowflakes.org • website: www.snowflakes.org

Started by Nightlight Christian Adoptions, the Snowflakes Embryo Adoption Program aims to place unused frozen embryos into adoption with qualified couples. It believes that life begins at conception and encourages couples that have undergone fertility treatments to place their unused frozen embryos into adoption as an alternative to donating them to research.

Society for Developmental Biology (SDB)
9650 Rockville Pike, Bethesda, MD 20814-3998
(301) 571-0647 • fax: (301) 571-5704
website: http://sdb.bio.purdue.edu/index.html

The purpose of the SDB is to further the study of development in all organisms and at all levels, to represent and promote communication among students of development, and to promote the field of developmental biology. On its website, the society provides links to publications regarding stem cell research.

Bibliography

Books

Kay Elder and Brian Dale, eds.	*In Vitro Fertilization*. New York: Cambridge University Press, 2000.
Geraldine Lux Flanagan	*Beginning Life*. New York: Dorling Kindersley, 1996.
Sarah Franklin	*Embodied Progress: A Cultural Account of Assisted Reproduction*. New York: Cambridge University Press, 1997.
Ronald M. Green	*The Human Embryo Research Debates: Bioethics in the Vortex of Controversy*. New York: Oxford University Press, 2001.
Suzanne Holland, Karen Lebacqz, and Laurie Zoloth, eds.	*The Human Stem Cell Debate: Science, Ethics, and Public Policy*. New York: Cambridge University Press, 2000.
Asim Kurhak, Frank A. Chervenak, and José M. Carrera, eds.	*The Embryo as a Patient*. New York: Parthenon, 2001.
William J. Larsen	*Essentials of Human Embryology*. St. Louis, MO: Churchill Livingstone, 1998.
Paul Lauritzen, ed.	*Cloning and the Future of Human Embryo Research*. New York: Oxford University Press, 2001.
M.J. Mulkay	*The Embryo Research Debate: Science and the Politics of Human Reproduction*. New York: Cambridge University Press, 2001.
R.G. Rosden	*Designing Babies: The Brave New World of Reproductive Technologies*. New York: W.H. Freeman, 1999.
Lauren J. Sweeny	*Basic Concepts in Embryology: A Student's Survival Guide*. New York: McGraw-Hill, 1998.
Alan O. Trounson and David K. Gardner, eds.	*Handbook of In Vitro Fertilization*. Boca Raton, FL: CRC Press, 2000.
Christopher Vaughan	*How Life Begins: The Science of Life in the Womb*. New York: Times Press, 1996.

Periodicals

John Entine and Sally Satel	"Inserting Race into the Stem Cell Debate," *Washington Post*, November 9, 2001.
John Garrey	"Is Nothing Sacred? What's Missing in the Stem Cell Debate," *Commonweal*, September 14, 2001.

Scott Gottlieb
"Adult Cells Do It Better," *American Spectator*, June 5, 2001.

James Greenwood
and Sam Brownback
"Symposium (Stem Cell Research)," *Insight on the News*, October 29, 2001.

Eric Juengst and
Michael Fossel
"The Ethics of Embryonic Stem Cells—Now and Forever, Cells Without End," *JAMA*, December 27, 2000.

Paul Lauritzen
"Neither Person nor Property: Embryo Research and the Status of the Early Embryo," *America*, March 26, 2001.

Laurie McGinley and
Antonio Regalado
"New Theory Could Roil Stem-Cell Debate," *Wall Street Journal*, August 3, 2001.

Gautam Naik
"Therapeutic Cloning Holds Promise of Treating Disease," *Wall Street Journal*, April 27, 2001.

National Catholic Reporter
"Stem Cells Hold Promise of Cures," October 22, 1999.

New York Times
"Downside of the Stem Cell Policy," August 31, 2001.

Wesley J. Smith
"The Good News You'll Never Hear: The Politics of Stem Cells," *National Right to Life News*, April 2001.

Gretchen Vogel
"Can Adult Stem Cells Suffice?" *Science*, June 8, 2001.

George Weigel
"Stem Cells and the Logic of Nazis," *Los Angeles Times*, September 3, 2000.

Robert J. White
"Do Human Embryos Have Rights?" *America*, June 19, 1999.

Index

abortion
  fetal tissue obtained from, 47
  legalization of, 48
  memorials for fetuses after, 18–19
  opposition to, and support for
    embryonic research, 37–38
  therapeutic cloning and, 42
Abuljadaye, Ilham, 65
adoption, embryo, 68–70, 71
adult stem cells
  corporate interest in, 64
  vs. embryonic stem cells, 10–12, 37
  potential of, 36–37, 52, 64–65
Advanced Cell Technology (ACT), 5, 42,
  43, 44
A.I. (film), 58
Anastrom Biosciences, 64
animals
  cloning, 55
  donor organs from, 41
  killing, vs. killing humans, 30
  mixing genomes across species and,
    43–44

blastocysts. *See* embryos
blood stem cells, 7
Boisseller, Brigitte, 57
bone marrow, fetal, 51
Bush, George W., 5, 36, 46

cadavers. *See* human cadavers
Callahan, Daniel, 13
cell therapies, 9
Center for Bioethics and Human
  Dignity, 45
China, 55–56
Clinton, Bill, 43, 47
cloning
  animals, 55
  ban on, 57
  humans, 42, 57
  see also therapeutic cloning
cryopreservation, 68
Cummins, Joe, 61
Cunningham, Randy, 37

Davidson, JoAnn L., 67
Deutsch, Peter, 55
disease, age-related degenerative, 39–40
DNA, 43–44, 59
Dolly (cloned sheep), 55

drug development, 8–9

embryonic stem cell research
  alternatives to, 51–53
  vs. animal experimentation, 34
  as beneficial, 8–10, 40
  debate over, 4–5
  destruction of potential person from,
    32
  enormous promise of, 12
  ethical considerations for, 42–43
  extravagant claims made about, 56–57
  federal funding for, 45
    ban on, support for not lifting, 70
    under George W. Bush, 46
    need for, 38
    opposition to, 53, 71
    rationale for, 46–47
    support for, 5
  Golden Rule applied to, 32–34
  guidelines sought for, 44
  horrific results from, 55–56
  is scientifically questionable, 50–51
  is unethical, 48–50
  laws against, 70–71
  mixing genomes across species and,
    43–44
  opposition to, 45–46, 70
  potential and value of, 36–37
  pro-life supporters of, 37–38
  standard argument against, 29–30
  vs. use of adult stem cells, 10–12
  violates existing law and policy, 46–48
  see also therapeutic cloning
embryonic stem cells
  vs. adult stem cells, 10–12, 37
  histocompatability problems of, 40–41
  sources of, 40, 62–63
  as unstable, 56
  see also pluripotent stem cells; stem
    cells
embryos
  acquisition of rights/interests, 34
  adoption from frozen, 68–70, 71
  baseline requirements for treatment of,
    21–22
  capacity to feel pain, 34–35
  frozen, 69–70
  from in vitro fertilization, 67–68
  gamete sources of
    connection to, 20–21

right of control by, 21, 22
as human beings, 4, 26–27, 38, 48–49,
  58–60
  con, 5, 27–29
laws protecting, 46, 47–48
moral respect for, 13–18, 23–24
questions on, 23
restrictions on treatment of, 22–23
vs. stem cells, 50–51
see also embryonic stem cells
Eshoo, Anna, 55
European Group of Ethics in Science
  and New Technologies (EGE), 64

Food and Drug Administration (FDA),
  41

Gearhart, John, 8, 62
Geron Corporation, 63
Goldstein, Lawrence S.B., 36

Hare, R.M., 32
Harkin, Tom, 71
Hatch, Orrin, 37, 38
hematopoietic stem cells, 51
Ho, Mae-Wan, 61
human beings
  cloning, 42, 57
  embryos as, 4, 26–27, 38, 48–49, 58–60
    con, 5, 27–29
  as having a right to life, 29, 30–32
  as indispensable, 58
human cadavers, 19–20
Human Embryo Research Panel, 47, 49

Infertility Clinic (University of Korea),
  63
Infertility (Medical Procedures) Act
  (1984), 34
In Vitro Fertilisation Committee, 34
in vitro fertilization
  controversy over, 4
  vs. embryo adoption, 68
  embryos for stem cell research received
    from, 7–8, 62
  first use of, 4
  frozen embryos from, 67–68
  Golden Rule applied to, 32–33
  increase in, 67
  process, 4

King, Nina, 57
Krauthammer, Charles, 54
Kuhse, Helga, 26

Lofgren, Zoe, 55

Mack, Connie, 37
McCain, John, 37

Meyer, Michael J., 13
mizuko kuyo rituals, 18–19
multipotent stem cells, 7, 62
  see also adult stem cells; embryonic
    stem cells

Nadler, Jerrold, 55
National Academy of Sciences, 57
National Bioethics Advisory
  Commission (NBAC), 43, 45, 46–47,
  49
National Institutes of Health, 6
National Neurological Institute and
  Stem Cell Research Institute, 65
Nelson, Lawrence J., 13
neural stem cells, 51–52
Nexell Therapeutics, 64
nuclear transfer. *See* therapeutic cloning

organs for transplantations, 9
Osiris Therapeutics, 64

Pelosi, Nancy, 55
pluripotent stem cells, 40
  defined, 7, 62
  vs. embryonic stem cells, 10–12
  vs. embryos, 50–51
  potential applications of, 8–10
  sources of, 7–8
  see also embryonic stem cells

reproductive cloning, 41–42

Singer, Peter, 26
Smith, Gordon, 37
Snowflakes Program, 68, 69–70
somatic cell nuclear transfer (SCNT). *See*
  therapeutic cloning
stem cells
  alternative sources of, 51–52
  commercial interests in, 63–64
  defined, 7, 46, 61–62
  vs. embryos, 50–51
  sources of, 37, 60
  see also adult stem cells; embryonic
    stem cells; pluripotent stem cells
Sullivan, Andrew, 58

therapeutic cloning
  banned, 54
  as beneficial, 9–10
  vs. cloning of human beings, 42
  destruction of embryos from, 63
  difficulties of, 55
  false hopes for, 54–55
  opposition to, 64, 65–66
  perceived advantage of, 62–63
  problem on source of oocytes for, 42
  process of, 41, 52–53

purpose of, 5
stem cells developed from, 8
in the United Kingdom, 41–42, 64
Thomson, James, 7–8, 62
Thurmond, Strom, 37
totipotent stem cells, 7, 8, 40, 61

United Kingdom, 41–42, 64
University of Korea, 63
U.S. Department of Health and Human
  Services (HHS), 5, 45, 46, 50, 51

U.S. Supreme Court, 48

Verfaillie, Catherine, 65

Waller Committee, 34
Warren, Mary Anne, 14
West, Michael D., 39
Wolf, Naomi, 19

zygote, 27
  see also embryos